MCQs for GP with Detailed Answers

BY: MORGAN PATEL

University Hospital Lewisham 2017

Preface

Whilst studying for Finals it was hardly believable the number of textbooks, notes, lectures and other resources that were available to satiate even the most demanding of student. An unhealthy culture of panic buying was almost encouraged, such was the vast amount of information that was expected and required.

However, with such an impressive armament at our fingertips it seemed illogical that there were few avenues for those diligent (or just plain lucky) enough to have accrued sufficient knowledge to want to put it to the test. Question books often provided coverage of topics likely to be encountered in examinations but often left frustration when incorrect choices were not explained.

This question book containing detailed answers was designed to address this need for explanation of not only the correct choice, but also why the other choices were incorrect, thereby providing the reader with positive feedback based on current medical practice. With 450 questions, based across 24 commonly tested areas of medicine, surgery and subspecialities and divided into five practice examination papers covering a mixture of subjects, MCQs provides a comprehensive review of these topics as well as providing exposure to frequently encountered question formats to help engender familiarity with examination styles.

PAPER 1

Multiple choice questions (single best answer)

1 A 75-year-old gentleman is referred by his GP to a consultant cardiologist for management of his newly diagnosed atrial fibrillation (AF). Palpitations and occasional shortness of breath are the only symptoms he has noticed and he has no past history of cardiovascular disease, but has suffered a transient ischaemic event in the past. On examination he is found to have an irregular heart rate ranging between 70 and 90 beats per minute and ECG confirms AF. Which of the following is the most appropriate next stage in his management?

a. Start digoxin for rate control.

b. Warfarinise the patient to reduce the risk of thromboembolism formation.

c. Start a beta blocker for associated hypertension.

d. Organise an echocardiogram.

e. Refer back to GP as his case can easily be managed in the community.

2 A 38-year-old gentleman attends A&E at 9 p.m. during a busy medical take. He complains of chest pain which has intermittently been present since the morning. On further questioning his pain is central in location with no radiation and some associated nausea. His father suffered with an MI at the age of 65 and his grandfather suffered from peripheral vascular disease. His troponin I is 0.05 (significant 0.1) and ECG shows no ischaemic changes. This gentleman asks you what happens next, what should you tell him?

a. He needs to be admitted for further bloods tests.

4

b. He requires an exercise tolerance test before he is discharged.

c. An echo will be useful in his further management.

d. He can be safely discharged without further follow-up.

e. He should be started on aspirin.

3 An 84-year-old nun presented to A&E 2 weeks after discharge from hospital under the care of the cardiologists. Her presenting complaint is one of feeling faint and dizzy and intermittently short of breath. She mentions that during her last admission she was started on digoxin because she had an irregular heart rate that was racing away. On discharge she claims that she had no problems and only developed this dizziness in the past couple of days. Her drug history includes atenolol 100 mg once daily. Her ECG today shows a rate of approximately 40 beats per minute with no association between P waves and QRS complexes. What is the next step in her management?

a. Insert a temporary pacing wire.

b. Give regular atropine.

c. Start amiodarone 200mg tds.

d. Stop atenolol.

e. Take bloods including drug levels.

4 A 69-year-old man was admitted from A&E 3 days after suffering a myocardial infarction. He was complaining of increasing shortness of breath and on observation was tachypnoeic at rest whilst sitting up. On examination he had no peripheral signs of disease, his jugular venous pressure was raised, he was breathing at 30 breaths per minute and his heart rate was 120/minute.

On auscultation there was evidence of a systolic murmur but no other findings. An erect chest X-ray was normal. Which of the following complications of MI is most likely to be the cause of this gentleman's shortness of breath?

a. Ventricular septal defect.

b. Recurrent infarction.

c. Aortic regurgitation.

d. Heart failure.

e. Dressler's syndrome.

5 A 45-year-old teacher was referred to the cardiologists after having been admitted with shortness of breath. Her past medical history consists of inflammatory bowel disease but no cardiac problems. On examination her apex was located in the anterior axillary line in the sixth intercostal space. There were no peripheral signs of cardiovascular disease but on auscultation a fourth heart sound was audible. There were no murmurs. Bedside 2D echo showed a dilated heart with an ejection fraction of 20– 25%. The likely cause of her dilated cardiomyopathy is:

a. Viral.

b. Alcohol.

c. Outflow obstruction.

d. Congenital.

e. Autoimmune.

6 The most appropriate diagnostic investigation in a patient presenting with chest pain and a widened mediastinum is:

a. 4 limb blood pressure measurements.

b. LFT's.

c. Lateral chest x-ray.

d. CT chest.

e. ECG.

7 A 16-year-old man presents to hospital complaining of abdominal pain, nausea and vomiting. He has been feeling unwell for the last 3 days since he

'caught a cold' from his younger sister.

His past medical history is remarkable only for childhood eczema and type I diabetes mellitus. He is in pain and unable to eat or drink anything because of pain in his stomach. Urine dipstick was taken that showed protein , ketones , glucose .

Which of the following insulin regimens should this man be

started on?

    a. Normal subcutaneous insulin with hourly blood glucose monitoring.

    b. Sliding scale of insulin with hourly blood glucose monitoring.

    c. Constant insulin infusion with hourly blood glucose monitoring.

    d. Change of normal insulin regimen to once daily long-acting insulin.

    e. Increase of normal insulin regimen to double requirements.

8 A 78-year-old woman is brought to accident and emergency from the warden-controlled accommodation where she resides. She was found in her apartment by the warden sitting on the floor and very confused. Past medical history is remarkable for pernicious anaemia, type II diabetes and vitiligo. On examination she is disorientated and scores 3/10 on the abbreviated mental test (AMT). Her abdomen feels lumpy and she is bradycardic at 50 beats a minute with a blood pressure of 152/92 and hypothermic at 34.9°C. Blood glucose was 4.1 mmol/L. Which of the following investigations is most likely to reveal the diagnosis?

    a. Thyroid function tests.

    b. Electrocardiography (ECG).

    c. CT scan of the head.

    d. Echocardiography.

    e. Short synacthen test.

9 Which of the following associations is correct?

a. Acute glaucoma – low intraocular pressure.

b. Conjunctivitis – conjunctival vessels do not blanch on pressure.

c. Iritis – dilated pupil.

d. Subconjunctival haemorrhage – hazy cornea.

e. Acute glaucoma – fixed, dilated pupil.

10 A 53-year-old man presents to his GP with a 2-week history of headache and recent blurred vision. He has been having the headaches at more frequent intervals in the past week and describes them as a 'tight band' around his head. Fundoscopy is performed, which reveals arteriolar narrowing and cotton-wool spots. Some oedema of the optic disc is also reported. Which of the following conditions is this fundoscopic appearance consistent with?

a. Diabetic retinopathy.

b. Hypertensive retinopathy.

c. Age-related macular degeneration.

d. CMV retinitis.

e. Ankylosing spondylitis.

11 Which area of the breast is most commonly affected by breast cancer?

a. Upper outer quadrant.

b. Upper inner quadrant.

c. Lower outer quadrant.

d. Lower inner quadrant.

e. Retro-areolar.

12 Risk factors for breast cancer include all of the following EXCEPT:

a. Nulliparity.

b. Late pregnancy 30 years.

c. Early menarche.

d. Late menopause.

e. High dietary dairy intake.

13 A 43-year-old man presents to his GP with a 1-week history of a painful swollen left knee. On examination the left knee is painful in all ranges of movement and is warm to touch.

There is evidence of a boggy diffuse swelling and routine blood tests reveal a neutrophilia, raised white cell count and pyrexia.

Which of the following investigations is the most important to perform?

a. Blood cultures.

b. Joint aspiration.

c. Serum urate levels.

d. MRI knee.

e. Skyline views of the knee.

14 A 23-year-old man presents to hospital with back pain and trouble performing at his basketball practices. On examination the only positive findings are of a reduced range of movement in back flexion and tenderness over the

left Achilles tendon.

Which of the following diagnoses is correct?

a. Early-onset rheumatoid arthritis.

b. Left-sided prolapsed lumbar disc.

c. Right-sided prolapsed lumbar disc.

d. Ankylosing spondylitis.

e. Facet-joint arthritis.

15- A 35-year-old man is admitted to the intensive care unit with respiratory failure secondary to a fungal chest infection. His past medical history reveals acute myelogenous leukaemia, splenom-egaly and a recent bone marrow transplant. His blood results reveal neutropenia and anaemia. Which of the following should be avoided unless absolutely necessary?

a. Respiratory system examination.

b. Abdominal and rectal examination.

c. Regular suction of nasopharyngeal secretions.

d. Daily bloods taken via a central venous catheter.

e. Regular turning to avoid pressure sores.

16- A 31-year-old vegan attends her GP practice complaining of fatigue. The GP is concerned about her dietary content and requests blood tests. She complains of no other symptoms and denies having heavy menses or any bleeds rectally. The GP is concerned about iron deficiency anaemia. Which of the following is not a recognised sign of iron deficiency anaemia?

a. Koilonychia.

b. Angular stomatitis.

c. Dysphagia.

d. Peripheral neuropathy.

e. Tongue atrophy.

17 A 10-year-old boy presents to A&E with abdominal pain and fatigue. The onset of the pain has been acute over the past 6 hours and is generalised. On further questioning he has no previous abdominal pathology and no clinical findings on examination. A family history reveals a cousin who suffers from sickle cell disease. Which of the following clinical features is NOT consistent with a diagnosis of sickle cell disease?

a. Pallor.

b. Splenomegaly.

c. Bone pain.

d. Leg ulcers.

e. Gallstones.

18 A 54-year-old man is brought to hospital by a concerned neighbour after finding him collapsed at home having taken an overdose of medication. He is assessed by the admitting house officer who elicits a history of suicidal ideation, a recent loss of appetite and lack of enjoyment of usual hobbies. The case is discussed with the duty psychiatrist who advises on further management. Which of the following statements regarding depression is NOT true?

a. Endogenous depression is more easily treated than exogenous (reactive depression).

b. Females are more likely to take a medication overdose as mode of suicide than males.

c. Lack of a confiding relationship is associated with depression.

d. Antidepressant medication takes action after approximately 2 weeks.

e. Thyroid disease should always be considered in the differential diagnosis of depression.

19 A 24-year-old man is brought in to hospital by a concerned neighbour after he is found trying to break into an electronics shop as he believed the government was using the television sets to control him. He is agitated on arrival to hospital and is demands to be released saying that it is all part of the government conspiracy keeping him hostage in hospital. He is persuaded to be admitted under the on-call team, however, you are called later than night by the nurse to assess him as he was found by the hospital security trying to escape. Which of the following is the correct course of action?

a. Admission to hospital under Section 3 of the Mental Health Act.

b. Cuff and restraint under common law.

c. Admission to hospital under Section 5(2) of the Mental Health Act.

d. Documentation of discharge from hospital against medical advice.

e. Discharge with community psychiatric follow-up.

20 Whilst carrying out an abdominal examination for a patient admitted with chest pain you notice a pulsatile and expansile mass in the abdomen. Upon mentioning it to the patient he confirms that he has been told in the past that he has an abdominal aortic aneurysm (AAA). He adds that he is under yearly surveillance and that it doesn't cause him any problems at present.

Which of the following statements about abdominal aortic aneurysms is INCORRECT?

a. More common in males than females.

b. 10% have associated popliteal aneurysm.

c. A diameter 4cm requires operative intervention.

d. Renal failure is a known postoperative complication of AAA repair.

e. There is a 5% risk of rupture when aneurysm reaches 6cm diameter.

21 A 64-year-old man presents with a urinary tract infection that has been unresponsive to a 5-day course of antibiotics started by his GP. Further questioning reveals he has suffered with problems with his chest for the last 10 years that he attributes to smoking since he was in his 20s. On examination he has a barrel-shaped chest, there is evidence of use of the accessory muscles of respiration and pursed lip breathing. Which of the following routine blood results is most likely to be found in this patient?

a. Lymphopaenia.

b. Anaemia.

c. Raised MCV.

d. Polycythaemia.

e. Thrombocytopenia.

22 A 69-year-old man was admitted from A&E 7 days after suffering a myocardial infarction (MI). He was complaining of increasing shortness of breath and on observation was tachypnoeic at rest sitting up. On examination, he had no peripheral signs of disease, his jugular venous pressure was raised, he was breathing at 30 breaths per minute and his heart rate was 120/minute.

On auscultation there was evidence of a systolic murmur but no other findings on examination. An erect chest X-ray was normal. Which of the following complications of MI is most likely to be the cause of this gentleman's shortness of breath?

a. Ventricular septal defect.

b. Recurrent infarction.

c. Aortic regurgitation.

d. Heart failure.

e. Dressler's syndrome.

23 A 7-year-old boy is referred by his GP to the on-call surgeons. He has attended the practice complaining of lower central abdominal pain and vomiting. The pain was acute in onset almost 2 hours prior to presentation but is gradually worsening. He notes that there have been similar episodes of pain in the past which spontaneously resolved themselves. He has no recent history of foreign travel or unusual diet. His temperature is 38.0°C and denies any diarrhoea. Examination of his ears, nose, throat and chest is normal. In this case which of the following must you be sure to check?

a. Rovsing's sign.

b. Scrotal examination.

c. Rectal examination.

d. Full blood count.

e. Abdominal X-ray.

24 Two hours after a football game in which a 34-year-old man was struck with the ball in the groin, he is brought to hospital with a swelling in the scrotum that has not resolved with application of an ice-pack. On examination there is a small scar in the right groin, the left testis is lying slightly higher than the right and there is a small, hard lump in the right testis. The testicular adnexae are firm but non-tender. These findings are suggestive of:

a. Torsion of the hydatid of Morgagni.

b. Epididymo-orchitis.

c. Seminoma.

d. Teratoma.

e. Scrotal haematoma.

25 A 31-year-old man presents to his GP complaining of an itchy rash on his hands. On questioning he reveals that he works for a Chinese restaurant in the back of kitchen as a dishwasher. On examination of his hands there are multiple excoriated sites on the dorsum and over the fingers of both hands with cracking of the skin over an erythematous base. The most likely diagnosis is:

a. Dermatitis.

b. Lichen planus.

c. Chemical burn.

d. Porphyria cutanea tarda.

e. Psoriasis.

26 A 38-year-old man presents to the dermatology clinic with intensely itchy elbows and knees. He states that this has been going on for the past 2 weeks and is interfering with his life to the point that he cannot take it any longer. Systemic enquiry reveals past episodes of malabsorption relieved by a wheat-free diet. He is not allergic to any medication and maintains a gluten-free diet. The most likely cause of his itch is:

a. Atypical eczema.

b. Psoriasis.

c. Dermatitis herpetiformis.

d. Scabies.

e. Polycythaemia rubra vera.

27 A 14-year-old girl presents to her GP distressed and upset. She tells you that she was in a relationship with an older boy and that they had been engaging in sexual intercourse. She had recently become worried that she was pregnant as they had been having unprotected sex and an over the counter pregnancy test confirmed this. She begs you not to tell her mother and to refer her to a family planning clinic for an abortion.

Which of the following is NOT the correct course of action?

a. Referral to a family planning clinic.

b. Counselling her about contraceptive options.

c. Offering her a sexually transmitted infection screen.

d. Informing her parents as she is a legal minor.

e. Advocating her discussing the pregnancy with her parents.

28 A 33-year-old lady presents to hospital on return from a ski-ing holiday. She is normally fit and well and describes an incident where her ski got caught in the snow causing her to fall over during which the ski did not release from her foot. She described immediate pain in her right calf which was then alleviated by simple analgesia. Examination and X-ray at the ski resort provide very limited help in a diagnosis. You are asked to see her and make a diagnosis of a ruptured tendo Achilles.

What would be your management plan?

a. Surgical tendo Achilles repair.

b. Above knee backslab.

c. Below knee cast with foot in neutral position.

d. Below knee cast with foot in equinus position.

e. Discharge with GP follow-up.

29 In patients with tibial plateau fractures which of the following nerves is most likely to damaged as a result of the injury?

   a. Common peroneal nerve.

   b. Tibial nerve.

   c. Sciatic nerve.

   d. Femoral nerve.

   e. Lateral cutaneous nerve of thigh.

30 A new non-invasive test for the influenza virus is produced by a pharmaceutical company based on a study of 1340 individuals. The data is published in an infectious disease journal that you are reading in your spare time and is given in table format below:

Test Disease

   Positive

Negative

Positive 580

150

Negative 140

450

Which of the following statements regarding statistical aspects of the new test is correct?

   a. The sensitivity of the test is (580/(580 140)) 80.1%.

   b. The positive predictive value of the test is 580/(580 140) 80.1%.

   c. There were 150 false negatives in the test.

   d. A high specificity will predict a low false negative rate.

   e. This test should be used as a screening test for influenza?

17

31 A 36-year-old multiparous woman presents to the emergency gynaecology unit after an episode of vaginal bleeding that was discovered after she was trying on some clothes in the maternity section of a department store. Further questioning reveals she is at 31 weeks' gestation, as confirmed by ultrasound scan. Her vital signs are BP 142/78, temperature 36.7°C, pulse 96/minute.

Which of the following is the most likely diagnosis?

a. Cervical cancer.

b. Placenta praevia.

c. Abruptio placentae.

d. Placenta accrete.

e. Chorio-amnionitis.

32 A 30-year-old primigravida who is 20 weeks pregnant contacts her midwife for advice about a painful right leg. She tells the midwife that the leg began to swell 2 days earlier and is now acutely painful to walk on. Clinically there is a discrepancy of 7 cm between the diameter of both calves. She has had no other problems during her pregnancy and there is no family

history of gestational problems. What is the likely diagnosis in her case?

a. Cellulitis.

b. Fat embolus.

c. Deep vein thrombosis.

d. Ischaemic limb.

e. Varicose veins.

33 A 4-year-old child is brought to his GP by his mother who is concerned about poor weight gain. He is at the 15th centile for height and weight and his past medical history includes admissions to hospital for recurrent chest

infections and an episode of gastroenteritis. Developmental parameters are normal except for slightly reduced hearing in the right ear, which is slightly erythematous. Which one of the following pathologies is likely in this child?

a. PAS positive macrophages on intestinal film.

b. Cobblestoned appearance on barium enema.

c. Single amino acid defect in a chloride channel transporter.

d. Double bubble on abdominal X-ray.

e. Abnormal bone marrow cytology.

34 An adolescent presents to his school doctor with bilateral tender and swollen breasts. He has become increasingly self-conscious of late and has been avoiding physical education classes.

On examination there are tender soft masses in the lower quadrants of both breasts. Which of the following is the most appropriate next step in managing this patient?

a. Urgent referral to social services.

b. Reassure the patient that this is normal.

c. Needle aspiration and send fluid for culture and cytology.

d. Referral to a breast surgeon for excision and biopsy.

e. Short course of oral prednisolone and 2-week review.

35 A 33-year-old gentleman presents with upper abdominal pain and vomiting. Blood tests demonstrate a raised white cell count and an amylase of 300 IU/L. Of the following differentials,

which is the LEAST likely to be correct?

a. Pancreatitis.

b. Perforated duodenal ulcer.

c. Ruptured abdominal aortic aneurysm.

d. Transverse colon diverticulitis.

e. Diabetic ketoacidosis.

36 Regarding clinical signs of abdominal disease, which of the following is associated with bowel perforation?

a. Rovsing's sign.

b. Murphy's sign.

c. Rigler's sign.

d. Kerr's sign.

e. Trousseau's sign.

37 A 55-year-old woman is 2 days post-fenestration of liver cysts. She is complaining of pain in the abdomen, nausea and malaise. Routine blood tests taken post-operatively show a bilirubin of 135 μmol/L, γ-GT of 210 IU/L, AST of 150IU/L with a slightly elevated WCC. Which of the following is the most likely explanation?

a. Biliary sepsis.

b. Propofol hepatotoxicity.

c. Common bile duct ligation.

d. Bile leak.

e. Cholecystitis.

38 A 65-year-old obese woman underwent an open cholecystectomy for

complicated gallstone disease 5 days ago. You are called to see her on the wards as she has become dyspnoeic, irritable and complaining of pain. Observations record a blood pressure of 110/60, pulse 66 and regular and saturations of 94% on 2L of oxygen. Her past medical history is of ischaemic heart disease and hypertension treated with daily aspirin, atenolol, simvastatin and frusemide. Which of the following post-operative complications is the most likely diagnosis?

a. Pulmonary embolus.

b. Post-operative atelectasis.

c. Myocardial infarction.

d. Left ventricular failure.

e. Diaphragmatic injury.

39 Which of the following is LEAST useful in investigating the above complication?

a. Computed tomography with pulmonary angiography (CT-PA).

b. Fibrin degradation product (D-dimer).

c. Arterial blood gas.

d. Electrocardiogram.

e. Chest radiograph.

40 A 53-year-old man presents to accident and emergency complaining of a warm, tender swelling in the right groin associated with nausea, vomiting and constipation. On examination there is a tender, 2 cm swelling that is irreducible. The decision for theatre is made and examination intra-operatively the relations of the mass are defined as medial to the inferior epigastric artery and above the

inguinal ligament. Which of the following correctly describes this mass?

    a. Spigelian hernia.

    b. Indirect inguinal hernia.

    c. Direct inguinal hernia.

    d. Femoral hernia.

    e. Ventral hernia.

41 A 37-year-old lady is admitted to hospital with what the A&E doctors suspect is a SEVERE asthma attack. Which of the following signs or symptoms is consistent with that diagnosis?

    a. Silent chest, peak expiratory flow rate (PEFR) 33% of predicted.

    b. Tachycardia 110/minute, PEFR 50% of predicted.

    c. Exhaustion, hypotension.

    d. PCO_2 normal or high on arterial sampling.

    e. Completing sentences, respiratory rate 15/minute.

42 A 57-year-old lady is seen complaining of acute onset shortness of breath. She is known to suffer from asthma, which is normally well controlled. Regularly she takes inhalers, both bronchodilators and inhaled steroids. She hasn't suffered an exacerbation of her asthma for a number of years and has never had any ITU admissions. Which of the following is NOT a reasonable differential diagnosis of an acute asthma attack?

    a. Anaphylaxis.

    b. Pneumothorax.

c. Upper respiratory tract obstruction.

d. Massive pulmonary embolus.

e. Upper respiratory tract infection.

43 A 25-year-old woman presents to accident and emergency after a sudden onset of shortness of breath. She has a past medical history of asthma and dysmenorrhoea. She denies any current medication apart from the oral contraceptive pill since her menarche. On examination she is a tall thin woman who is tachypnoeic with a pulse of 122. BP is 94/56 with a raised JVP.

ECG demonstrates sinus tachycardia. Which of the following treatments is the most appropriate?

a. Carotid massage with cardiac monitoring.

b. Needle aspiration in the second intercostal space anterior chest.

c. Slow i.v. frusemide infusion.

d. Nebulised bronchodilators.

e. Low molecular weight heparin.

44 A 34-year-old man is brought in by his colleagues with acute dyspnoea following an office summer party. Regular medications include salbutamol inhaler and over the counter antihistamines for allergic rhinitis. On examination there is evidence of stridor and some peri-oral swelling. What is the most important next step in managing this patient?

a. Nebulised salbutamol.

b. Intramuscular adrenaline.

c. Intravenous hydrocortisone.

d. Insertion of a laryngeal mask airway.

e. Endotracheal intubation.

45 A 22-year-old man is brought in to hospital following a high-speed road traffic accident where he was the driver. On initial assessment he is found to be drowsy with marked facial injury, chest injury consistent with steering wheel impact and multiple areas of subcutaneous emphysema. He is tachycardic with respiratory distress and further respiratory examination reveals a displaced trachea to the left side of the chest. Which of the following is the first step in management?

a. Endotracheal intubation.

b. Needle thoracocentesis of the right chest.

c. Insert a nasopharyngeal airway.

d. Insert a chest drain with underwater seal.

e. Perform an emergency tracheostomy.

46 A 63-year-old gentleman presented to casualty with chest pain and shortness of breath. He described the chest pain as right sided and intermittent. The pain and shortness of breath were exacerbated by deep respiratory effort but ameliorated by shallow breathing. He has no risk factors for coronary artery disease. He has a past medical history of severe Parkinson's disease and is cared for by his wife. He takes levodopa and carbidopa but no other medications. On examination he has inspiratory crepitations at the right base but no other findings. Which of the following is the most likely cause for his symptoms?

a. Atypical pneumonia.

b. Aspiration pneumonia.

c. Reflux disease.

d. Levodopa toxicity.

24

e. Parkinson's disease associated heart failure.

47 A 16-year-old girl presents to accident and emergency having taken 35 paracetamol tablets that morning. She is tearful and upset and history taking is difficult as she does not answer questions easily. Her past medical history is of depression and self-harm and childhood eczema. Examination is unremarkable and blood tests reveal an Hb of 10.8, slightly low albumin with normal urea and electrolytes. AST, bilirubin, γ-GT, alkaline phosphatase and ALT are normal. INR is 1.12 with a fibrinogen less than 6 and a normal APTT. Which of the following investigations is the most sensitive indicator of hepatic damage?

a. AST and ALT.

b. Alkaline phosphatase.

c. INR.

d. Fibrinogen.

e. Albumin.

48 A 68-year-old woman is admitted to the ward after an elective hip replacement for osteoarthritis. On post-operative day 3 her respiratory function starts to deteriorate and she starts to complain of profuse diarrhoea. A sputum sample is obtained and sent off to the laboratory and appropriate antibiotic therapy commenced. Four days later she is dehydrated with reduced skin turgor. Recent blood results show moderately low potassium, high urea and a stool culture result pending. Which of the following steps is appropriate in managing this patient?

a. Administration of i.v. potassium at a rate of 20mmol/hour.

b. Administration of oral metronidazole.

c. Administration of oral amoxicillin.

d. Administration of 2 units of blood.

25

e. Administration of a potassium sparing diuretic.

49 A 23-year-old woman presents to hospital feeling nauseated, unwell, with loss of appetite. She tells you that this occurred over a month and she was very worried she was pregnant as she had missed her last period. Further questioning reveals no recent history of travel, she drinks two or three glasses of wine a week and has been married for 2 years. Systemic review reveals a 2-week history of a painful right knee that happened after falling whilst ice skating. On examination she is comfortable at rest but has a mild yellow tinge to the sclera and an itchy rash over her forearm. The abdomen is very tender over the right upper quadrant but Murphy's sign is negative. Which of the following diagnoses is most likely?

a. Viral hepatitis.

b. Budd–Chiari syndrome.

c. Cholecystitis.

d. Autoimmune hepatitis.

e. McArdle's disease.

50 A 63-year-old man presents to his GP with a month's history of regurgitating food, foul-smelling breath and a sensation of gur-gling in her neck when he eats. He describes the regurgitated food as slightly changed but denies any blood or pain when he eats. He has not lost any weight recently and says that apart from the symptoms described he is otherwise fit and well.

Which of the following diagnoses is most likely?

a. Pharyngeal pouch.

b. Plummer–Vinson syndrome.

c. Chagas' disease.

d. Oesophageal carcinoma.

e. Mallory–Weiss tear.

51 A 34-year-old man with ulcerative colitis presents in the gastroenterology outpatient clinic with abdominal pain and fatigue.

He states the pain has been intermittent for the past 2 weeks and has not settled with simple analgesia. Focussed questioning reveals that the pain is distinct from that of his ulcerative colitis flare-ups and he has not experienced any change in bowel habit recently. Routine blood tests taken prior to clinic show a markedly raised alkaline phosphatase with mild hyperbilirubi-naemia. Haemoglobin is slightly reduced but the rest of the blood tests are normal. Which of the following would be the most appropriate next investigation?

a. CT scan of the abdomen.

b. Endoscopic retrograde cholangiopancreatogram (ERCP).

c. Colonoscopy.

d. Plain abdominal radiograph.

e. Liver biopsy.

52 A 52-year-old man presents to hospital complaining of abdominal pain and diarrhoea. He has had 10 bouts of diarrhoea since the morning and states that the pain is severe. He has noticed that his bowels have become much more watery over the past 2 months and that he has been increasingly breathless. Recently he has stopped taking alcohol as he has noticed that on occasion his face and neck become violently red and he feels hot and nauseated and attributes this to drinking red wine. On examination he is slightly anxious and breathless whilst lying flat. There is peripheral pitting oedema of the ankles and abdominal examination reveals a 3cm smooth but tender hepatomegaly. Cardiac sounds are abnormal with a pansystolic murmur and a raised jugular

venous pressure. Which of the following investigations is likely to be most useful diagnostically?

  a. 24-hour urine protein collection.

  b. Plasma osmolality.

  c. 24-hour urine 5-hydroxyindoleacetic acid (5-HIAA).

  d. Urinary osmolality.

  e. 24-hour urine for 4-hydroxymethoxymandelate (VMA).

53 A 26-year-old man was admitted by ambulance suffering with severe headaches. He described the headaches as the worst pain he had ever experienced and mentioned that concurrently he felt unsteady and drunk. He described the pain as being occipital in location and of rapid onset, being continuous with a duration of up to a minute. He has no relevant past medical or family history of note and works as a truck driver. On examination; he is apyrexial, GCS 15/15 there are no focal neurological signs. What is the next step in investigation of this gentleman's headache?

  a. MRI brain.

  b. CT scan of head.

  c. Lumbar puncture.

  d. Blood cultures.

  e. Admit for neurological observations and regular analgesia.

54 Relatives of a 70-year-old lady were concerned that she appeared to be increasingly confused. On examination she was orientated in time, place and person but did have slurred speech.

Further neurological examination revealed bilateral past pointing and trunkal ataxia with no evidence of nystagmus. Routine blood tests revealed no cause for these symptoms. Where is this lady's lesion most likely to be located?

a. Bilateral basal ganglia.

b. Left temporo-parietal lobe.

c. Cerebellar vermis.

d. Left lateral cerebellar lobe.

e. Left-sided frontal lobe.

55 A 70-year-old gentleman who is known to be taking warfarin is admitted to hospital with left-sided weakness. He has a history of coronary artery disease for which he is taking the warfarin but examination reveals no other findings of note. Which of the following investigations is the most important to obtain?

a. Carotid duplex scan.

b. Echocardiogram.

c. CT scan of the brain.

d. INR.

e. ECG.

56 A 24-year-old lady presents with progressive seizure-like jerking movements of all extremities. She has three siblings all of whom are normal; although a cousin was thought to have suffered with a similar illness and died prematurely at the age of 37 years. No diagnosis was made for her cousin. On admission her GCS was 15/15, although she was slightly confused. A CT scan of her brain was normal but a follow-up MRI scan revealed areas of reduced density bilaterally at the basal ganglia. Routine blood tests revealed deranged liver function tests but nothing else of note. Which of the following is the most likely diagnosis?

a. Early-onset Parkinson's disease.

b. Wilson's disease.

c. Glycogen storage disorder.

d. Porphyria.

e. Lead poisoning.

57 A 50-year-old man presents to his GP with headache, tenderness over the scalp and a general feeling of being tired all the time. Focused questioning reveals he also suffers with muscular aches and feels he has been a bit slow of late. Routine bloods were sent off and a 2-week appointment is made to review the results. Which of the following diagnoses is LEAST likely in this man?

a. Superficial temporal arteritis.

b. Migraine.

c. Tension headache.

d. Viral meningitis.

e. Cluster headache.

58 A 30-year-old woman was admitted to casualty with a 24-hour history of worsening headaches. She described the headaches as constant with no relieving factors and associated nausea but on direct questioning she confirms that the pain is exacerbated by strong light. On examination there are no peripheral neurological signs but you note papilloedema on fundoscopy. Which of the following options is not a cause of this sign?

a. Meningitis.

b. Benign intracranial hypertension.

c. Cerebellar haemangioblastoma.

d. Hyperparathyroidism.

e. Malignant hypertension.

59 A 54-year-old man presents feeling unwell with a failure to pass urine for 24 hours. Blood results taken on admission show a raised urea and creatinine and his blood pressure lying is 165/92.

Abdominal palpation reveals a suprapubic dome-shaped mass that is dull to percussion. CT scan of the abdomen reveals a poorly defined peri-aortic mass and a bladder volume estimated to be 1.5L. Which of the following drugs are most likely responsible for this presentation?

a. Gold.

b. Paracetamol.

c. Acyclovir.

d. Rosiglitazone.

e. Methysergide.

60 A 46-year-old woman recently returned from visiting her relatives in Bangladesh. Shortly after her return she developed a fever, became unwell and complained of an ache in her left flank. Detailed questioning reveals a 7k weight loss since her return 3 weeks ago and diarrhoea that has been manifest on and off over the same period. On examination she is tender in the renal angle and a mid-stream urine result demonstrates a sterile pyuria. What is the next step in management for this woman?

a. Treat for a fungal pyelonephritis.

b. Treat empirically with a 7-day course of antibiotics.

c. Intravenous urogram.

d. Chest X-ray.

e. Cystoscopy.

Extended matching questions

Chest pain

a. Acute MI.

b. Pneumonia.

c. Pulmonary embolus.

d. Pericarditis.

e. Bornholme's disease.

f. Pneumothorax.

g. Gastro-oesophageal reflux disease.

h. Aortic dissection.

Select the most suitable option for each of the scenarios below: 61 An 87-year-old female nursing home resident has started to complain of chest pain. There are no exacerbating or relieving factors for the pain. The nurses note that she is also short of breath. She suffers with chronic obstructive pulmonary disease which is usually well controlled on inhaled medications.

62 A 30-year-old secretary who has recently recovered from viral chest infection presents to A&E with intermittent chest pain.The chest pain is central in origin with no radiation or any associated symptoms. On examination the chest pain is recreated by exerting gentle pressure on the sternum.

63 A 68-year-old gentleman has complained of retrosternal chest pain. He notes that it is at its worse in the early afternoon and evening. The pain does not wake him from sleep but is recreated when he lies flat. He complains of

associated nausea but no vomiting. He takes regular aspirin for coronary artery disease and has recently had a short course of diclofenac for joint pains.

64 A 58-year-old gentleman is brought in to A&E by ambulance following an episode of chest pain at work. His colleague that accompanied him to the hospital mentioned that he described central chest pain which felt like it as tearing through to his back.

65 One week following a total knee replacement a 63-year-old woman starts to complain of chest pain. It is right sided in location and exacerbated by inspiration. It has no radiation or associated symptoms. She had previously complained of a swelling in her right calf which was thought to be related to her joint replacement.

Manifestations of endocrine disease

a. Cushing's syndrome.

b. Acromegaly.

c. Diabetes mellitus.

d. Diabetes insipidus.

e. Phaeochromocytoma.

f. Syndrome of inappropriate ADH secretion (SIADH).

g. Hypothyroidism.

h. Hyperthyroidism.

The following patients have all presented with endocrine disease.

Please choose the most likely diagnosis from the list above. Each option can be used once, more than once or not at all.

66 A 54-year-old man presents to the renal clinic for regular follow-up post-live-related kidney transplant. He complains of a feeling of lethargy, weight gain and has been complaining of swelling of his ankles recently. There is no

tenderness at the site of renal transplant and ultrasound demonstrates no abnormality. Blood pressure reading is 176/98 with a fasting blood glucose level of 10.2 g/dL. Blood results show a sodium of 148 mmol/L with a potassium of 3.5 mmol/L.

67 A 78-year-old woman is brought to hospital by her neighbour who is concerned that she has become confused recently. On examination she is alert but not orientated in time or place and is noted to be tired and uncooperative during physical examination. Abdominal examination reveals a lumpy quality to the abdomen and areas of erythema ab igne on both shins. A keen medical student notes some unusual hair loss over her eyebrows and scalp.

68 A 52-year-old man presents to hospital with shortness of breath and cough productive of green sputum. He complains that he has been feeling weak, thirsty and thinks his high blood pressure medication may be at too high a dose as he has been urinating frequently for the past week and has lost a significant amount of weight over the last month. Past medical history is remarkable for hypertension. Chest radiography confirms a lower respiratory tract infection. Blood results reveal a sodium of 147 mmol/L, potassium of 4.9 mmol/L, urea of 11 mmol/L with a plasma osmolality of 330 mOsm/L. Urine osmolality is verbally reported as being 'high'.

69 A 42-year-old man presents to his GP for a yearly check-up offered in his area. His past medical history is unremarkable and he states that aside from some recent changes in his vision and headaches, both of which he attributes from some new glasses he bought a few weeks ago he feels well. On examination he is a tall and heavy set man who is very tanned from a recent holiday. Cardiovascular, respiratory and abdominal examination is unremarkable but you notice an area of untanned skin around his left ring finger and he tells you regretfully that recently his wedding band has become too tight and is being resized.

70 A 38-year-old man presents to his GP complaining of recurrent anxiety attacks. He describes three or four episodes whilst he has been out in public of feeling light-headed with palpitations and a mild tremor that causes him to want to sit down until the feeling subsides. Focussed questioning reveals he has become constipated recently and he is very anxious that this may be cancer as his family have a history of 'renal and pancreatic growths'.

Rheumatological conditions

a. Gout.

b. Rheumatoid arthritis.

c. Osteoarthritis.

d. Pseudogout.

e. Septic arthritis.

f. Ankylosing spondylitis.

g. Polymyalgia rheumatica.

h. Psoriatic arthropathy.

The following patients have all presented with rheumatological problems. Please choose the most correct diagnosis from the above list. Each option may be used once, more than once or not at all.

71 A 27-year-old girl presents to her GP with pain and swelling in her joints, particularly the small joints of the hands. She has noticed this discomfort for the past month but has no other symptoms other than a bit of malaise and non-specific feeling of 'not being herself'. She had put these symptoms down to having a young child. She takes the combined oral contraceptive pill but no other medications and suffers with no other illnesses.

72 A 47-year-old builder complains of pain in his foot. On examination there is evidence of redness and discomfort in the right hallux although there is no evidence of ulceration or skin changes. Social history reveals an intake of alcohol in the region of 40 units/week, often in binges, and a diet rich in red meat.

73 A 63-year-old lady returns to the rheumatology clinic with pain in the joints of the hands and some loss of function. The ring finger on her right hand has become shortened in length, all other fingers are normal although there is a degree of ulnar deviation. Current medications include topical steroids, tar and regular light therapy.

74 A 23-year-old man presents to his GP with an increasing pain in his lower back and stiffness that is worse in the mornings.

He has noticed some intermittent pain in his knees and increasing pain in the soles of his feet towards the end of the day.

Spine X-ray reveals squaring of the vertebrae.

75 A 74-year-old lady has suffered with increasing pain in her hip for a number of years, which she tolerates with NSAIDs. Recently she has noticed squaring of the thumb joint on her left hand and the pain in her hip is becoming more problematic and more troublesome towards the end of the day.

Opportunistic infections in HIV/AIDS

a. Pneumocystis jerovici pneumonia.

b. Candidiasis.

c. Toxoplasmosis.

d. Cryptosporidium infection.

e. Cryptococcal infection.

f. Varicella zoster pneumonitis.

g. Cytomegaly virus infection.

h. Mycobacterium avium intracellulare.

The following HIV positive patients have all presented with opportunistic infections. Please choose the most correct diagnosis from the above list. Each option may be used once, more than once or not at all.

76 A 34-year-old man presents to hospital with abdominal pain, crampy in nature and associated with loose watery stools. On examination he is pale, tachycardic and sweaty. He denies eating any seafood recently but had been staying at a friend's farm for the past 2 weeks.

77 A 40-year-old woman presents to hospital with a 3-day history of headache, nausea, lack of appetite. She has been otherwise fit and healthy and describes the headache as not related to any particular time of day but associated with pain on looking at bright lights.

78 A 28-year-old woman presents to her GP with pain on swallowing solid food and a strange taste in her mouth. She describes the pain as retrosternal in nature and associated only with swallowing; worse with dry and solid food and less with liquids. She denies any significant weight loss.

79 A 45-year-old man is brought to hospital by his friends who are worried that he has been acting 'out of character' recently.

Collateral history reveals a gradual change in his behaviour, becoming more confused and agitated over a 2-month period with an episode of shaking of the limbs and arms that was attributed to medication side-effects. On arrival to accident and emergency he is aggressive, disruptive and would not allow any of the nursing staff to take blood from him.

80 A 32-year-old man was found collapsed at home by his partner and brought by ambulance to accident and emergency. On arrival he is struggling to breathe and is on an oxygen mask. History from the partner reveals a gradual onset over the past 2 weeks of increasing shortness of breath and feeling of tiredness after the simplest of tasks. On examination he is tachypnoeic with a respiratory rate of 34 breaths a minute and on auscultation fine crepitations are heard in the lower and midzones of the lungs.

Treatment of psychiatric disorders

a. Olanzipine.

b. Sertraline.

c. Cognitive behavioural therapy.

d. Electroconvulsive therapy.

e. Eye movement desensitisation and reprocessing.

f. Temazepam.

g. Reduction in caffeine intake.

h. Lithium.

The following patients have all presented with a psychiatric disorder. Please choose the most appropriate treatment modality from the above list. Each option may be used once, more than once or not at all.

81 A 34-year-old woman is brought to hospital by a friend who is concerned that recently she has been acting bizarrely; going on shopping trips every other day and spending money in the local betting shop, which she never used to do. She has also been socialising more often than usual and had been throwing house parties every weekend.

82 A 42-year-old aid worker presents to his GP with 5-week history of inability to sleep, a feeling of being on edge and easily startled and nightmares of persecution and violence. He had previously returned from an aid mission overseas where he had to be evacuated due to unsafe conditions.

83 A 24-year-old man who has recently arrived in the United Kingdom is referred to the acute psychiatric clinic by his GP who is concerned that he has been experiencing auditory hallucinations telling him that the immigration officials have been monitoring his activities and are planning to use him as a spy.

He become agitated when confronted about these thoughts and claims that people are stealing ideas from his head.

84 A 43-year-old woman presents to her GP complaining of feeling a sense of overwhelming fear associated with shortness of breath and a racing heart beat when she is asked to give a presentation or speak in front of lots of people. She says that the thought of having to do any kind of social activity makes her feel nauseated.

85 A 67-year-old woman is brought to accident and emergency by her neighbour who has been increasingly worried about her behaviour. She is unkempt and was found by her neighbour at home in her chair where she had

not moved for 3 days. She has been on antidepressant medication in the past started by her GP. Psychiatric assessment in hospital revealed a low mood with deep suicidal ideation and morbid delusions.

Diseases of the hand

a. Dupuytren's contracture.

b. Glomus tumour.

c. Paronychia.

d. Nailbed haematoma.

e. Radial nerve injury.

f. Lower brachial plexus root injury.

g. Carpal tunnel syndrome.

h. Scaphoid fracture.

The following patients have all presented with diseases of the hand. Please choose the most likely diagnosis from the above list.

Each option may be used once, more than once, or not at all.

86 A 35-year-old keen gardener presents to her GP with a swollen left index finger. She states that it has caused her throbbing pain for the past 2 weeks and came on after she cut her finger on some rose thorns. There is swelling, redness and tenderness surrounding the nail itself on the left index finger only.

87 A 43-year-old man presents with an extremely painful mass under one of the nails of his right hand. He states that he has become more aware of the mass over the past month. There is a bluish hue to the mass with lifting of the nailbed.

88 A 31-year-old woman is brought in to accident and emergency after cutting herself with a knife following a break-up with her partner. On examination of her hand there are multiple lacer-ations on the wrist by the base of the thumb. She complains of an inability to extend her wrist.

89 A 13-year-old boy falls onto concrete whilst roller-skating. He is seen by the out of hours GP and is found to have a tender swollen base of the thumb with tenderness in the anatomical snuffbox. He has weakness on making a pincer grip but has normal abductor pollicis brevis function.

90 A 54-year old man who is seen regularly in the endocrinology clinic presents with the complaint that during the night he wakes up with tingling and numbness in his hands that is only relieved by shaking them out. On further questioning he has otherwise been fit and well but states that in recent years he has gone up many shoe sizes and cannot now fit into his favourite hat.

PAPER 2

Questions

Multiple choice questions (single best answer)

1 A 27-year-old man is referred from accident and emergency on a Friday night. He is complaining of pain in his left hand and describes injuring it by punching a wall following a fight with his girlfriend. He notes that the hand is swollen and he is not quite able to form a fist due to the pain and swelling. Neurovascular supply is intact. On X-ray you note a mid-shaft fifth metacarpal fracture that appears to be rotated on the true lateral view. How would you manage this case?

a. Below elbow backslab and fracture clinic follow-up.

b. Sling for support and outpatient physiotherapy.

c. Admit for open reduction and internal fixation of fracture.

d. Admit for analgesia and physiotherapy.

e. GP review in 1 week.

2 A 58-year-old gentleman was admitted complaining of lower back pain. He noted that the back pain had gradually worsened and had now stopped responding to analgesia. He described some radiation of the pain into his right thigh but denied any sciatica-like symptoms. He was afebrile and had a limited straight leg raise to 30 degrees. Hip movements were good bilaterally. X-rays of his lumbar spine revealed no cause for his symptoms. His past medical history includes angina and a pneumonectomy 9 months earlier for a malignant mesothelioma. Which of the following investigations will provide the best diagnostic information?

a. Blood cultures.

b. Bone scan.

c. MRI spine.

41

d. Lumbar puncture.

e. CT spine.

3 A 14-year-old boy is brought to hospital by ambulance having been involved in a road traffic accident. He was in the front seat and was wearing a seatbelt but had been incorrectly belted. He arrives intubated by the ambulance crew and is hypotensive.

A FAST scan demonstrates free fluid in the abdomen from a ruptured spleen. He is scheduled for emergency surgery for exploratory laparotomy and splenectomy. As he is being taken to theatre his parents arrive from home and demand that he not be given any blood transfusions as he is a Jehovah's Witness and show you their cards stating so. Which of the following actions is the correct course of action?

a. Refuse to proceed to surgery without blood.

b. Proceed to surgery using crystalloid replacement only.

c. Proceed to surgery as an emergency using blood as necessary.

d. Reschedule surgery to allow for auto-transfusion.

e. Apply for a court order to allow surgery to proceed.

4 A young child is brought to her GP by her mother who has noticed she has developed a rash over her face and neck. The child is otherwise well and the mother describes no other symptoms apart from a mild itch that occurs now and again around the lesions. On examination there are multiple small pearly papules with a central umbilicated area of keratin plug distributed randomly over the face and neck. Which of the following is most likely to be the cause of this rash?

a. Varicella zoster virus (VZV).

b. Herpes simplex virus (HSV).

c. Molluscum contagiosum.

d. Eczema.

e. Pityriasis versicolor.

5 A 34-year-old man is referred from the surgical team and seen by the dermatologists for an itchy rash in his elbow creases, which he has been scratching for the past week. He is diagnosed with eczema on inspection of the rash. Which of the following patterns is NOT part of the eczema classification?

a. Atopic eczema.

b. Asteatotic eczema.

c. Discoid eczema.

d. Arthropathic eczema.

e. Varicose eczema.

6 A 72-year-old Afro-Caribbean man presents to his GP after problems initiating micturition. He has taken to wearing a pad during the day and finds that he has to use the toilet frequently at night, with occasional urinary accidents and post-void dribbling.

Abdominal examination is remarkable only for a fullness in the lower abdomen and routine blood tests, urea and electrolytes are normal. The next best step in management is:

a. Suprapubic catheterisation.

b. Blood glucose.

c. Anti-dsDNA antibody.

d. Prostate-specific antibody.

e. Ultrasound scan of the renal tract.

7 A 54-year-old man presents feeling unwell with a failure to pass urine for 24 hours. Blood results taken on admission show a raised urea and creatinine

and his blood pressure lying is 165/92 mmHg. Abdominal palpation reveals a suprapubic domeshaped mass that is dull to percussion. CT scan of the abdomen reveals a poorly defined peri-aortic mass and a bladder volume estimated to be 1.5 L. Which of the following drugs are most likely responsible for this presentation?

a. Gold.

b. Paracetamol.

c. Acyclovir.

d. Rosiglitazone.

e. Methysergide.

8 A fit 26-year-old lady was admitted to hospital with cellulitis of her left leg later found to be secondary to a spider bite. She was started on intravenous antibiotics – flucloxacillin and benzylpenicillin having no known drug allergies. The on-call house officer was called to see her due to the nurse noticing some facial flushing. On further questioning she admitted to suffering with tingling in her hands and teeth but no shortness of breath or chest tightening. She remained apyrexial throughout. What would be your next course of action?

a. Consider this to be an anxiety attack and continue treatment with reassurance.

b. Add in erythromycin as current cover is not adequate.

c. Change antibiotics due to allergy.

d. Stop antibiotics, administer steroids and antihistamines.

e. Continue treatment with topical antibiotics.

9 A 79-year-old lady with known chronic obstructive pulmonary disease has been admitted 6 times in the past 6 months. On this admission she complains of increasing shortness of breath and difficulty in coping at home. On observation from a distance this lady is comfortable at rest with a respiratory rate of 14/minute. At the bedside, observation reveals a tachypnoea and breathing through pursed lips. Arterial blood gas studies for assessing

domiciliary oxygen requirements are found to be negative and this has been the case on previous admissions.

Physiotherapists have noted that her mobility is good. Your team decides that she is medically fit for discharge, what will be your next step?

a. Continue rehabilitation at a local cottage hospital.

b. Ask social services for review with nursing home placement in mind.

c. Keep patient in hospital until she feels ready to leave.

d. Send her home with a GP follow-up immediately.

e. Impress on the patient that she is well and that she has no medical problems requiring attention.

10 A 97-year-old lady is referred to the on-call surgical team by her GP. She has been complaining of a cold, painful leg for the past 6 hours. On examination the GP notes that the skin appears to be mottled and notes the absence of pulses below the femoral artery on the affected side. Of note her past medical history includes arrial fibrillation for which she is not anticoagulated. On examination she is noted to have a respiratory rate of 35/minute and evidence of bibasal inspiratory crepitations which chest X-ray confirms as bilateral pneumonia. What diagnosis was the GP concerned about in this lady?

a. Buerger's disease.

b. Femoral artery embolus.

c. Arterial insufficiency.

d. Abdominal aortic aneurysm.

e. Venous ulceration.

11 A 32-year-old woman presents to her GP complaining of recurrent episodes of intense discomfort associated with shortness of breath, chest pain and palpitations usually whilst she is out in public places. The episodes last between 5 and 10 minutes are usually cease on their own. Her past medical history is unremarkable but she tells you that her family have a history of 'heart attacks' and is worried that her symptoms may be related. Which of the following associations is NOT true?

a. Irritable bowel syndrome.

b. Agoraphobia.

c. Mitral valve prolapse.

d. Chronic obstructive pulmonary disease (COPD).

e. Age over 65 years.

12 A 43-year-old man presents to clinic with feelings of a lack of enjoyment of his usual hobbies, a feeling of detachment from his family and friends associated with poor sleep, nightmares and irritability. He describes these changes happening a few months ago and states that he has been easily startled and ill at ease ever since. His past medical history is remarkable only for allergic rhinitis and a recent hospital admission for a head injury following a robbery at his home. Which of the following diagnoses is the most likely?

a. Acute stress disorder.

b. Depressive disorder.

c. Post-traumatic stress disorder (PTSD).

d. Schizoid personality disorder.

e. Generalised anxiety disorder (GAD).

13 A 5-year-old girl is brought to her GP by her mother as she is worried about her health. She has always been a well child until recently when she has become increasingly tired and pale. Her mum is concerned that she intermittently suffers with fevers that are not well controlled with paracetamol. She has now gradually developed a rash and the main concern is one of bacterial meningitis. On clinical examination she does not appear to be acutely unwell. She has noticeable pallor of the conjunctiva and has a widespread purpuric rash which blanches on pressure. The GP advises a paediatric review and some blood tests which show low platelet count and a leukopaenia. What is the likely diagnosis in this case?

a. Bacterial meningitis.

b. Acute lymphocytic leukaemia.

c. Chronic myeloid leukaemia.

d. Acute myeloid leukaemia.

e. Viral encephalitis.

14 Which of the following facts about chronic leukaemia is INCORRECT?

a. CLL is a chronic incurable condition.

b. Ionising radiation is a known cause of CML.

c. CLL cells contain the Philadelphia chromosome.

d. Early disease prognosis for CLL is 8–10 years.

e. CLL is a malignant disease of B-lymphocytes.

15 A 42-year-old man presents to his GP with a 2-month history of a painless lump in his neck. He has noticed this lump grow slowly bigger and as he had been feeling tired with sweats at night he had thought it was lymph node from a 'head cold'.

Recently he has noticed that he cannot enjoy wine or beer anymore because they cause him pain. Which of the following diagnoses is the most likely?

a. Hodgkin's lymphoma.

b. Infectious mononucleosis.

c. Non-Hodgkin's lymphoma.

d. Polycythaemia rubra vera.

e. Myelodysplastic syndrome (MDS).

16 A 51-year-old woman presents to accident and emergency with episodes of coughing up blood over a 2-week period. Further questioning reveals a history of weight loss, frequent cough and a feeling of tiredness and malaise. Routine blood tests taken in hospital reveal an erythrocyte sedimentation rate of 70 mm/hour, Sodium of 135 mmol/L, Potassium of 5.3 mmol/L,

creatinine of 167 µmol/L, urea of 9.3mmol/L, with a mild neutrophilia and haemoglobin of 10.2 g/dL. Which of the following investigations is most likely to be positive?

a. c-ANCA.

b. Anti-glomerular basement membrane.

c. Anti-SCL 70.

d. Anti-mitochondrial antibodies.

e. Rheumatoid factor.

17 A 48-year-old former secretary, known to the rheumatologists, presents to clinic with a 2-week history of tingling over her fingers and hands and numbness over the palms of her fingers and thumbs apart from the little fingers

on both hands.

On examination there are multiple bilateral joint deformities and tapping over the volar aspect of the wrist exacerbates the symptoms described above. Which of the following treatment options should be considered next?

a. Intra-articular steroid injection.

b. Carpal tunnel decompression.

c. Nerve conduction studies.

d. Plain radiographs of both wrists/hands.

e. Wrist splinting.

18 Optimal assessment of a breast lump in a 55-year-old lady is best described by which of the following?

a. Clinical examination, ultrasound and biopsy.

b. Clinical examination and mammogram.

c. Ultrasound, mammogram and biopsy.

d. Clinical examination, mammogram and biopsy.

e. Clinical examination, chest X-ray and biopsy.

19 A 31-year-old lady is referred by her GP as she is complaining of breast pain. She is 1-week post-partum and has been breast feeding but it has now become too painful to continue. The GP notes that on examination there is evidence of a collection in one of the breasts with overlying erythema and associated pain. An ultrasound scan confirms an abscess. What is the most appropriate management?

a. Oral flucloxacillin.

b. Incision and drainage of abscess.

c. Needle aspiration.

d. Analgesia and cold compress.

e. Admit for i.v. antibiotics.

20 A 34-year-old woman who is under regular review in the rheumatology clinic is seen in accident and emergency with a urinary tract infection. Whilst in hospital she is examined by some medical students who notice that her vision in the right eye is poor with diplopia in the same eye. She has a history of cardiac problems and examination of the cardiac system reveals a soft diastolic murmur heard best in the aortic area. Which of the following diagnoses would this clinical picture be most consistent with?

a. William's syndrome.

b. Down's syndrome.

c. Marfan's syndrome.

d. Turner's syndrome.

e. Reiter's syndrome.

21 A 64-year-old woman is seen by her GP for a very red, itchy and painful eye. She describes the eye as having the sensation of there being a bit of 'grit stuck in it'. When she is asked about these symptoms she says she has had these symptoms on and off for a long time but never this badly. On further enquiry she suffers from a dry cough and has trouble eating very dry food as she finds it 'sticks to her mouth and is difficult to swallow'.

Which of the following diagnoses is the most likely?

a. Anterior uveitis.

b. Acute glaucoma.

c. Subconjunctival haemorrhage.

d. Sjögren's syndrome.

e. Retinal vein occlusion.

22 A 69-year-old man with type II diabetes mellitus is brought to hospital with confusion, drowsiness and aggressive behaviour.

He lives with his daughter who noticed that he had become 'not himself' and had checked his blood sugar, finding it to be 2.3 mmol/L. Which of the following are NOT associated with hypoglycaemic states?

a. Liver failure.

b. Gliclazide.

c. Insulinoma.

d. Addison's disease.

e. Cushing's disease.

23 A 58-year-old woman presents to the thyroid clinic to have a check-up for long-term hypothyroidism for which she is taking thyroxine 100 μg once daily. She tells you in the clinic that she has read about a novel therapy for thyroid disease that doesn't involve tablets and would like to try this if possible. Her blood results are available in the clinic and demonstrate a high thyroid stimulating hormone and a high T4. Which of the following is most likely to explain these results?

a. Subclinical hypothyroidism.

b. Sick euthyroid syndrome.

c. Non-compliance and overdosing prior to clinic.

d. Inadequate replacement with thyroxine.

e. Over-replacement with thyroxine.

24 Mid-ward round a nurse asks you to review one of your well-known patients with acute onset shortness of breath. The nurse is concerned that the patient looks unwell and requests your opinion. You remember that the patient recently suffered an myocardial infarction, on assessment you note that the airway is patent but the patient is acutely short of breath. The first step in your management is:

a. Contact your senior colleagues for assistance.

b. Perform an arterial blood gas.

c. Attach a cardiac monitor.

d. Request a chest X-ray.

e. Complete a primary survey.

25 Which of the following is not a clinical finding associated with infective endocarditis?

a. Osler's nodes.

b. Retinal haemorrhages.

c. Splinter haemorrhages.

d. Clubbing.

e. Erythema nodosum.

26 An 84-year-old gentleman was given an urgent outpatient cardiology appointment by his GP. He was concerned about the increasing swelling of his legs and his shortness of breath. On examination he was able to walk with sticks but oedema had spread up to his groin. He was notably short of breath and on auscultation he had bibasal inspiratory crepitations up to the midzones. He is currently on digoxin for a history of arterial fibrillation and other medications include furosemide 40 mg once daily. You are asked to admit the patient, what changes will you make to his medications?

a. Add in bumetanide.

b. Change furosemide to i.v. and double the daily dose.

c. Add an ace inhibitor.

d. Start a beta-blocker.

e. Add in metolazone.

27 A 35-year-old lady attended accident and emergency with chest pain. She had no history of cardiovascular disease and denied any risk factors. Blood tests showed a positive troponin and ECG showed antero-lateral ischaemic changes. Which of the following illegal drugs are associated with this presentation?

a. Amphetamines.

b. Cocaine.

c. Cannabis.

d. Heroin.

e. Rohypnol.

28 A patient on the coronary care unit is a 30-year-old lady. Your

consultant suggests that you examine her as she has interesting findings. As you look over you notice that she is a tall slim lady wearing glasses. What would you expect to find on auscultation?

a. Systolic murmur at the right upper sternal edge.

b. Diastolic murmur at the right upper sternal edge.

c. Systolic murmur at lower left sternal edge.

d. Systolic murmur at the apex.

e. Diastolic murmur at the apex.

29 In patients newly diagnosed with arterial fibrillation on digoxin therapy, which of the following electrolytes is most important to monitor?

a. Serum sodium.

b. Serum potassium.

c. Serum calcium.

d. Serum magnesium.

e. None of the above.

30 A 54-year-old man presents to hospital with lethargy, shortness of breath and complaining of itching all over. His previous notes state he is well known to the renal physicians for chronic renal failure secondary to diabetic nephropathy and is followed up in the joint diabetic/renal clinic regularly. History taking reveals he has been having a lot of trouble recently for arthritic pain in his hip and has been taking some pain medication from the chemists. On examination there is bilateral pitting oedema to the mid-thigh and he is short of breath with a respiratory rate of 30 breaths a minute. Oxygen saturations are at 87% on room air. He provides a list of the current medications he is taking. Which of the following medications has most likely precipitated this admission?

a. Erythropoietin.

b. Frusemide.

c. Ibuprofen.

d. Pioglitazone.

e. Chlorpheniramine.

31 A 10-year-old boy is brought to hospital by his mother who is worried that he has passing very dark smoky urine. She states that this started this morning and has been intermittent over the course of the days. She is also worried that his face has become more swollen over the last couple of days and he has not been feeling himself. On further questioning the mother tells you that he had been fine up until a nasty bout of 'flu' that he caught from school just over a week ago that required a few days off school. Which of the following diagnoses is the most likely?

a. Minimal change glomerulonephritis.

b. Post-streptococcal glomerulonephritis.

c. Henoch–Schönlein purpura.

d. Berger's disease (IgA nephropathy).

e. Rapidly progressive glomerulonephritis.

32 A 54-year-old man with chronic renal failure is seen at his regular follow-up with his GP. Blood pressure is taken showing a reading of 145/78 mmHg with a normocytic anaemia, Hb 9.5 g/dl, urea of 11.4 mmol/L and a creatinine of 145 μmol/L. Which of the following is NOT associated with chronic renal failure (CRF)?

a. Anorexia.

b. Nausea.

c. Restless legs.

d. Hypokalaemia.

e. Hyperphosphataemia.

33 A 43-year-old woman presents to hospital with shortness of breath, malaise and bilateral pitting oedema to the knees. She is treated for acute renal failure and started on a diuretic that acts at the thick ascending limb of the loop of Henlé. Which of the following diuretics acts at this particular site?

a. Acetazolamide.

b. Mannitol.

c. Frusemide.

d. Bendrofluazide.

e. Spironolactone.

34 Which of the following states is NOT an indication for renal replacement therapy (dialysis)?

a. Refractory metabolic acidosis.

b. Oliguria.

c. Severe hyperkalaemia.

d. Uraemic symptoms.

e. Drug ingestion.

35 Whilst on your general practice attachment you are asked to pay a visit to an 81-year-old gentleman. His wife died 3 years earlier following a large myocardial infarction and since he has been managing at home independently. His daughter is concerned that he doesn't seem to be himself. She notes that he is becoming increasingly forgetful and on occasion doing strange things like leaving the taps running or the oven on when it is not in use. In the case of Alzheimer's disease, which of the following is incorrect?

a. A CT brain will be normal.

b. Dysphasia may be the presenting feature.

c. Brisk reflexes and upgoing plantars are often seen.

d. There may be relevant family history.

e. Depression is commonly seen.

36 A 31-year-old bank clerk presents to her GP complaining of the worst headache that she has ever experienced. On taking a history the GP elicits that this headache was acute in onset, sharp in nature and had no exacerbating or alleviating features. She denies any history of trauma. The patient notes that she is stressed at work and mentions a family history of migraines. She denies any nausea, vomiting, hallucinations or visual disturbances but notes that that headache is still present and showing no signs of improvement. Examination is unremarkable and observations are stable. Her past medical history includes dysmenorrhoea for which she takes the oral contraceptive pill but nil else of note. The GP refers her to the on-call medical team for review. Which diagnosis is he particularly concerned about?

a. Bacterial meningitis.

b. Tension headache.

c. Subarachnoid haemorrhage.

d. Subdural haemorrhage.

e. Benign raised intracranial pressure.

37 A 48-year-old woman presents to hospital complaining of vomiting and diarrhoea. The symptoms started in the early hours of the morning after a staff conference. She denied eating any seafood or drinking any alcohol but states that she did eat the buffet food, which was chicken fried rice and vegetable spring rolls. On examination there are no physical signs apart from a previous lower segment Caesarean section in the abdomen.

Which of the following organisms is the most likely infectious agent?

a. Rotavirus.

b. Clostridium botulinum.

c. Cryptosporidium parvum.

d. Bacillus cereus.

e. Escherichia coli.

38 A 68-year-old woman with renal cell cancer presents to hospital with abdominal pain and abdominal distension. She states that her abdomen has been becoming more distended over a 3-week period with pain throughout this time. She also states that she was afraid to come into hospital as she thought this was further spread of the cancer. On examination she has a tender distended abdomen with 4-cm smooth hepatomegaly and evidence of fluid shift. The abdominal veins are dilated and there is evidence of caput medusae at the umbilicus. Which of the following diagnoses is the most likely?

a. Viral hepatitis.

b. Epstein–Barr virus infection.

c. α1-antitrypsin deficiency.

d. Wilson's disease.

e. Budd–Chiari syndrome.

39 A 26-year-old man presents to his GP with recent change in bowel habit, diarrhoea with mucous and blood-streaks and abdominal pain over a month period. He has also noticed that it has become very painful to pass stool to the extent that he sometimes resists the urge to defaecate until he can hold it no longer. Colonoscopy is arranged that shows multiple areas of cobblestone appearance and aphthous ulceration. Which of the following statements regarding this disease is correct?

a. Surgical therapy is likely to be curative.

b. Disease is limited to the terminal ileum and distally.

c. Transmural involvement is seen on histology.

d. Continuous inflammatory change is seen on colonoscopy.

e. Barium follow-through is of no use diagnostically.

40 A 23-year-old man presents to accident and emergency feeling lethargic, passing large amounts of urine and complaining of abdominal pain. He states that for the past 2 weeks he has had a cough and has been finding himself more breathless when walking to work. Past medical history is remarkable for type I diabetes mellitus and he is a smoker of 20 cigarettes a day. Urine dipstick done on admission show glucose ⧄⧄, ketones ⧄⧄⧄ and trace protein. Venous blood gases results show a pH of 7.29, bicarbonate of 18 mmol/L with a base excess of ⧄3.4 mmol/L. Which of the following treatment regimens should be instituted?

a. Double the usual basal bolus insulin regimen with strict blood glucose monitoring hourly.

b. Start short-acting insulin infusion with 5-L fluid replacement of 0.9% sodium chloride with potassium as required over a 24-hour period.

c. Add a long-acting insulin to the usual basal bolus regimen with 5-L fluid replacement with 0.9% sodium chloride.

d. Start short-acting insulin infusion to reduce blood glucose to less than 15 mmol/L then restart high-dose oralhypoglycaemic with strict blood glucose measurement.

e. Start a sliding scale of intermediate-acting insulin with 5-L fluid replacement of 0.9% sodium chloride with basal bolus short-acting insulin as required.

41 A 68-year-old woman presents with pain in her abdomen causing her to vomit. She states she has lost her appetite for food and can't hold anything down. Examination of the abdomen reveals localised tenderness over the left iliac fossa. Digital rectal examination reveals flecks of blood mixed with the stool.

Routine blood tests show a white cell count of 17.3 ⊠ 109/L, C-reactive protein of 110 mg/l, urea of 6.9 mmol/L and creatinine of 118 µmol/L. Which of the following is NOT an indication for surgery?

a. Faecal peritonitis.

b. Colovesical fistula.

c. Large bl obstruction.

d. Tender palpable mass.

e. Failure to exclude cancer.

42 A 43-year-old man with known alcoholic liver disease presents to hospital with a distended abdomen, pain and yellow discolouration to his skin and sclera. On examination of the chest there are multiple blanching red raised lesions over the upper torso and arms, and loss of chest and axillary hair distribution.

Abdominal examination reveals a 5-cm tender hepatomegaly with dilated tortuous veins around the umbilicus. Regarding portal-systemic venous anastomoses in portal hypertension,

which of the following associations is NOT correct?

a. Left gastric with azygous leading to oesophageal varices.

b. Paraumbilical with inferior epigastric leading to caput medusae.

c. Superior to middle/inferior rectal leading to rectal varices.

d. Splenic with left gastric leading to splenic varices.

e. Retroperitoneal and phrenic leading to diaphragmatic varices.

43 A 77-year-old man with known bibasal lung fibrosis is admitted to hospital for assessment of the need of long-term oxygen at home. He is already on home oxygen as required but his GP is concerned that he may need more regular therapy. Results of an arterial blood gas (ABG) taken on 35% oxygen via facemask are: pH 7.41, PO2 11.1kPa, PCO2 5.4kPa, bicarbonate 26mmol/

L. Which of the following is most appropriate in this case?

a. Reduce oxygen to 28% and repeat ABG.

b. Increase oxygen to 40% and repeat ABG.

c. 35% is adequate oxygen for this patient.

d. Increase oxygen to 60% and reassess.

e. Repeat ABG measurement on air.

44 Whilst working on a busy medical firm at a teaching hospital you are asked to take some medical students to see interesting cases in order to improve their examination skills. You take them to see a 76-year-old gentleman who has the following clinical signs: unilateral ↓ chest expansion, ↓ breath sounds and ↓ percussion note. Which of the following clinical conditions would provide these clinical signs?

a. Pneumothorax.

b. Fibrosis.

c. Consolidation.

d. Pleural effusion.

e. Extensive collapse/lobectomy/pneumonectomy.

46 Whilst on placement at your local GP practice you are asked to see a 78-year-old man who is complaining of shortness of breath. He has no history of respiratory disease and denies use of inhalers. On examination you note that he has a temperature of 38°C and auscultation findings are consistent with a right lower zone pneumonia. Which of the following is the commonest cause of a community acquired pneumonia?

a. Haemophilus influenzae.

b. Mycoplasma.

c. Moraxella catarallis.

d. Streptococcus pneumoniae.

e. Staphylococcus aureus.

47 Following making an accurate diagnosis of a community acquired pneumonia, which of the following antibiotics would you start as first-line treatment, bearing in mind that the patient has normal renal function and no

known drug allergies?

   a. Erythromycin.

   b. Cefalexin.

   c. Amoxicillin.

   d. Augmentin.

   e. Metronidazole.

48 Mr Roberts is a 70-year-old man who has recently returned from a Mediterranean holiday. Over the past few days he has felt like he has the flu. He has been suffering with muscle aches, fever tiredness and has now developed a dry cough. He is becoming increasingly short of breath and his chest X-ray shows a bibasal consolidation. His past medical history includes a myocardial infarction and type II diabetes which is diet controlled. He smokes 10 cigarettes a day. Which of the following organisms is most likely to be the cause of his problem?

   a. Legionella.

   b. Mycoplasma pneumoniae.

   c. Chlamydia pneumoniae.

   d. Pneumococcus.

   e. Staphylococcus aureus.

49 A young child presents with regurgitation of food and vomiting noticed by the mother to occur frequently after meals. She is worried that the child has failed to progress along the normal centile chart and finds that the vomiting is worse when the child lies horizontal after mealtimes. Further investigation reveals a moderate congenital diaphragmatic hernia. Which of the following statements regarding diaphragmatic hernias is correct?

a. Traumatic right-sided defects are more common than left-sided defects.

b. Large central hernias may present as respiratory distress in neonates.

c. Hernias through the foramen of Morgagni are usually significant.

d. Congenital hiatal hernias almost always require surgical treatment.

e. Traumatic diaphragmatic hernias are usually treated conservatively.

50 Regarding factors associated with peptic ulcer disease, which of the following is NOT considered to be a risk factor for ulceration?

a. Pregnancy.

b. Male sex.

c. Head injury.

d. Severe burns.

e. Steroids.

51 A 15-year-old boy is admitted for pain in the right iliac fossa associated with nausea and vomiting for 3 days with signs of peritonism. The diagnosis is made and the child taken to the operating theatre. Twelve hours post-operatively the nursing staff are worried as the child is vomiting. Blood pressure and temperature measurements are normal and urine output is good.

On examination the abdomen is soft but tender. According to the last entry in the notes he has been allowed to eat and drink but has not managed to keep anything down. Which of the following post-operative complications is most likely to have occurred?

a. Small bowel obstruction.

b. Anastomotic leak.

c. Adverse reaction to anaesthetic agent.

d. Acute stress ulceration.

e. Post-operative ileus.

52 On seeing the patient you arrive at a diagnosis and decide on further management of the vomiting. Which of the following options should be considered in the first instance?

a. Nasogastric tube insertion for oral intake.

b. Erect chest radiograph.

c. Abdominal radiograph.

d. Anti-emetic medication.

e. Proton pump inhibitor.

53 A 76-year-old man is referred from his GP to hospital due to recent weight loss, high blood glucose readings of 18 mmol/L and yellow discolouration of the skin and sclera. Routine blood tests reveal markedly deranged liver enzymes, normal urea and electrolytes, and normal full blood count. Examination reveals an obese habitus, yellow discolouration of the skin and sclera, and 5-cm non-tender hepatomegaly. Which of the following diagnoses is the most likely?

a. Pancreatic adenocarcinoma.

b. Cholangiocarcinoma.

c. Choledocholithiasis.

d. Hepatitis.

e. New-onset diabetes mellitus.

54 A 82-year-old man presents with progressive shortness of breath, paroxysmal nocturnal dyspnoea and orthopnoea over the past 3 weeks. Further questioning reveals a past medical history that is remarkable for osteoarthritis and right knee replacement. He is a heavy smoker and drinks moderate alcohol.

Clinical examination reveals tachypnoea, tachycardia and bilateral ankle swelling. Dullness of the percussion note of the right hemithorax is elicited with reduced vocal resonance as well as asymmetrical chest wall movement on inspiration. Auscultation reveals reduced breath sounds to the right midzone and bibasal crepitations. Which of the following should be carried out next?

a. Echocardiography.

b. Chest radiography.

c. Pleural tap and drainage.

d. Intravenous clarithromycin and amoxicillin.

e. Electrocardiogram.

55 A 13-year-old boy falls onto concrete whilst roller-skating. He is seen by the out of hours GP and is found to have a tender swollen base of the thumb with tenderness in the anatomical snuffbox. He has weakness on making a pincer grip but has normal abductor pollicis brevis function: Which of the following is the MOST LIKELY diagnosis?

a. Paronychia.

b. Nailbed haematoma.

c. Radial nerve injury.

d. Lower brachial plexus root injury.

e. Scaphoid fracture.

56 A 14-year-old girl presents to her GP with severe cramping abdominal pain and diarrhoea for the past 2 weeks. She had a similar episode 8 weeks earlier, which resolved without medical attention. At present the diarrhoea is bloody and bowel motions are associated with crampy abdominal pains. In addition the GP notes oral ulcers, which are painful and according to the patient have been present for the past 3 days. Her family history includes a grandfather who had a colostomy for a gastro intestinal (GI) problem. What is the most likely cause for her symptoms and signs?

a. Crohn's disease.

b. Ulcerative colitis.

c. Henoch–Schönlein purpura.

d. Shigella infection.

e. Giardia infection.

57 A 23-year-old lady has attended the accident and emergency department complaining of a high fever, diarrhoea and vomiting. She has noticed a headache and occasional muscle aches.

She has no past medical history of note and has had no recent illnesses. Her menstrual cycle is regular lasting for 5 days a month and her most recent period finished 5 days ago. On examination she appears dehydrated and is hypotensive. What is the most likely diagnosis in her case?

a. Viral gastroenteritis.

b. Bowel ischaemia.

c. Dysmenorrhoea.

d. Pregnancy.

e. Toxic shock syndrome.

58 Which of the following associations is incorrect?

a. Trichomonas – yellow discharge.

b. Chlamydia – chronic cervicitis.

c. Gonorrhoea – urethritis.

d. Gardnerella vaginalis – white discharge.

e. Atrophic vaginitis – yellow discharge.

59 In estimating the prevalence of disease in a small town, the public health statistician gathers population data including epi-demiological data regarding the number of cases and deaths over the past year. There are currently 20,000 people who suffer from the disease. There were 250 deaths over the past year attributed to the disease and 500 new cases were diagnosed in the same period. Information regarding deaths was further broken down into those occurring due to natural causes and those due to violent crime or homicide of which there were 135 and 28, respectively. The population of the town is estimated from voting records to be 140,000. Which of the following correctly describes the prevalence of the disease?

a. 250/20,000.

b. 500/140,000.

c. 500/20,000.

d. 20,000/140,000.

e. 250/140,000.

60 Which of the following is NOT a lower motor neurone cause of a facial nerve palsy?

a. Bell's palsy.

b. Acoustic neuroma.

c. Ramsay Hunt Syndrome.

d. HIV.

e. Cerebrovascular accident.

Extended matching questions

Hip pain

a. Irritable hip.

b. Fractured neck of femur.

c. Slipped upper femoral epiphysis.

d. Hip dislocation.

e. Peri-prosthetic fracture.

f. Congenital dislocation of the hip.

g. Perthes' disease.

h. Septic arthritis.

61 A 78-year-old overweight lady with a history of osteoarthritis of the right hip and a total hip replacement presents to accident and emergency. She tried to contact her GP but was unable to get an appointment. She is complaining of pain on the lateral aspect of her right leg and in her right groin, and has been unable to weight bear since the morning when she fell over and landed on her right hip. On examination you note that her leg is shortened and internally

rotated whilst being held in an adducted position. The neurovascular supply to the leg is intact.

62 A 7-year-old boy is referred by the GP to the orthopaedic team for hip pain which has gradually developed over the past 4 hours. His mother notes that over the same time period he has developed a limp and is not keen on moving his leg and is insisting on being carried everywhere. Plain X-rays show no obvious problem and an ultrasound of the affected hip shows a collection of fluid. He is afebrile and other wise well and his hip does not feel hot.

63 An 87-year-old gentleman was referred by the on-call general practitioner for review. He noted that the patient was a nursing home resident and had suffered a fall a week ago but was still complaining of right hip pain. During the past week he has been treated with regular analgesia and despite this has experienced difficulty in weight bearing due to pain. The on-call GP was asked to review the patient today due to worsening of his hip pain at rest and was reluctant to weight bear or mobilise on that leg. On examination the GP noted that his leg was found to be shortened and externally rotated with tenderness on palpation of the groin and greater trochanter. Straight leg raise was limited due to pain and internal rotation caused severe pain, all other hip movements were satisfactory.

64 A 49-year-old lady presents to accident and emergency 6 weeks after insertion of a hip resurfacing prosthesis. Since the operation she describes the hip as, 'not ever being quite right'. In the 2 days prior to presentation she noticed increasingly bad pain in her right hip (same side as prosthesis) which radiates into her groin. The pain is preventing her from weight bearing although whilst lying supine all hip movements are possible passively to some degree although they are limited by pain.

65 A 78-year-old man complains of left-sided hip pain. It has been present for the past 6 hours and is becoming increasingly painful to the point that he is unable to weight bear. His GP is called out to see him and notes a fever of 38°C with pain on palpation of the hip joint and virtually no movement in any direction

in the hip. He has a history of having a right total hip replacement 3 years ago. He is referred to the on-call orthopaedic team and blood results show WBC 17.1 * 109/L, CRP 56 mg/L, ESR 24 mm/hr. What is the likely diagnosis?

Substance abuse

a. Cocaine.

b. Amphetamines.

c. LSD.

d. Phencyclidine (PCP).

e. Benzodiazepines.

f. Opioids.

g. Alcohol.

h. Barbiturates.

i. Marijuana.

The following patients have all presented with signs and symptoms of substance abuse. Please choose the most likely substance of abuse from the above list. Each option may be used once, more than once or not at all.

66 A 43-year-old businessman presents to hospital after going for some drinks with colleagues from work. He is restless, stating that he doesn't need to be in hospital and asking when he can go home. On examination he is tachycardic at 120 beats per minute with dilated pupils. Whilst you are examining him he starts to have episodic chest pain.

67 A 52-year-old man is admitted to hospital as he was found wandering the streets confused and 'talking to himself'. He is well known to the local hospitals attending frequently with malnutrition and chest infections. On examination he has heavily injected conjunctiva, appears to be hearing voices and does not readily make eye contact. He is somnolent and exhibits a lack of interest in food or drink when brought to him.

68 A 62-year-old woman is brought to hospital having suffered a fall in the street. On arrival she is disorientated and complaining of chest pain. An ECG performed demonstrates a prolonged QT interval and U waves. On examination she exhibits a lateral gaze palsy and is very unsteady on her feet.

69 A 32-year-old woman is brought to accident and emergency found collapsed in a nearby residential estate. She is unconscious on arrival and paramedics are securing an endotracheal tube with 100% oxygen on arrival to hospital. Her blood pressure reading is 90/55 mmHg on her left arm and her temperature is 34.7°C. An arterial blood gas reading taken in hospital demonstrates a pH of 7.31 with a PO2 of 15kPa and a PCO2 of 6.3 kPa.

70 A 17-year-old high-school student is brought to hospital by his parents who were concerned about his recent strange behaviour. He was found in his room unable to move his legs and complaining that his room was all blurry. On arrival to hospital he is sweating, agitated and violent with a blood pressure of 195/89 mmHg. Neurological examination reveals no pyramidal abnormality but is remarkable for a florid vertical nystagmus.

Genitourinary discharge

a. Candidiasis.

b. Trichomonas vaginalis (TU).

c. Chlamydia trachomatis.

d. Lymphogranuloma venereum.

e. Haemophilus ducreyi.

f. Bacterial vaginosis.

g. Gonorrhoea.

h. Donovanosis.

The following patients have all presented with genitourinary discharge. Please choose the most correct diagnosis from the above list. Each option may be used once, more than once or not at all.

71 A 33-year-old secretary presents to her GP with an offensive discharge that she noticed 2 days ago. She initially thought it might have been related to her menstrual cycle, however she denies any previous episodes of discharge. A vaginal swab is taken when it is noticed that the discharge smells fishy, however, with a normal appearance to the vagina on speculum examination. Slide microscopy reveals the presence of epithelial clue cells.

72 A 23-year-old man presents to the sexual health clinic with discharge from the penis and a burning sensation on passing urine. He has never had an episode like this before and when questioned he admits to casual sex with multiple partners since breaking up with his girlfriend a month ago. On examination there is a yellowish discharge from the urethra and microscopy shows Gram-negative intracellular diplococci.

73 A 42-year-old man presents to his GP with on itchy rash on his penis. He denies any recent sexual intercourse and has not travelled out of the country for many years. He states he has had the rash for some time with no ill effect. On examination the head of the penis has multiple red lesions with cracked and raw skin. His past medical history is remarkable only for osteoarthritis and type II

diabetes mellitus treated with diclofenac and metformin.

74 A 34-year-old woman presents to her GP as she and her husband have been trying for their first child for the past year and a half. She is embarrassed and upset to talk about their sexual habits and is frustrated because all her sisters have borne children already. On further questioning she reveals that she used to work as a prostitute but has 'given that all up now'. An endocervical swab is taken and the organism grown from cell culture is reported as being an obligate intracellular bacterium.

75 A 45-year-old woman presents to her local general practice nurse appointment for a routine smear test. She has not been for regular appointments with the nurse before. Whilst performing the smear test the nurse notices that the surface of the cervix is dotted with small haemorrhages and that there is an offensive, frothy, yellow-green discharge in the vagina with multiple erythematous areas on the vaginal walls.

Seronegative arthritides

a. Reiter's syndrome.

b. Enteropathic arthropathy.

c. Rheumatoid arthritis.

d. Ankylosing spondylitis (AS).

e. Reactive arthritis.

f. Scleroderma.

g. Psoriatic arthropathy.

h. Enthesopathy.

The following patients have all presented with rheumatological problems.

Please choose the most correct diagnosis from the above list. Each option may be used once, more than once or not at all.

76 A 31-year-old businessman presents to his GP complaining of an ache in his right knee with an inability to weight bear for the past week. He denies any history of trauma and recent travel history is remarkable only for a 12-hour flight to Thailand a few weeks previously. He denies any previousepisodes of joint problems. On examination he is reluctant to remove his trousers when examining the knee and you notice he has a very tender, sore left eye.

77 A 53-year-old man presents to the rheumatology clinic for regular follow-up. He undergoes regular light therapy and his only medications are topical tar and ibuprofen for chronic back pain. On examination he has pitting of his nails on two of the digits on one hand with an asymmetrical oligoarthritis affecting the small joints of both hands.

78 A 20-year-old man presents with a pain in his left foot associated with walking and standing. He works in an office as a sales clerk and denies any particularly strenuous exercise recently.

On examination when asked to demonstrate the site of pain he has particular difficulty bending over to touch his foot. Further questioning reveals a similar episode of pain affecting the 'tendon at the back of his right ankle' last year.

79 A 22-year-old man presents to his GP with a 2-month history of pain and stiffness in his back, associated with a reduced range of movement. He noticed this whilst stretching before a football game. He is anxious during the consultation and tells you that he is worried as he has been experiencing a tight sensation around his chest associated with pain that sometimes happens in the morning. Schoeber's test is markedly reduced.

80 A 34-year-old woman presents to hospital with multiple episodes of loose stools associated with some mucous and blood. History taking reveals a history of weight loss, fluctuating diarrhoea and previous hospital admission for a severely painful red eye.

She has been investigated previously at her GP for back pain and swollen joints.

Abdominal pain

a. Intussusception.

b. Pyloric stenosis.

c. Hirschsprung's disease.

d. Volvulus.

e. Appendicitis.

f. Nephroblastoma.

g. Inguinal hernia.

h. Constipation.

81 A 9-year-old girl is brought to see the GP by her mother.

She has been complaining of passing heavily bloodstained urine, which her mother believes represents early menarche.On further questioning the girl also complains of left-sided abdominal pain that is constant but has gradually been worsening over the past few weeks. She denies any constitutional symptoms and generally feels well. On examination she has a mass in her left loin.

82 A 4-year-old boy is brought to the accident and emergency department by his worried father. He has noticed that his son appears to be generally unwell and seems to be adopting a ball-like position for comfort. He is denying abdominal pain. He has passed one stool that appeared to be quite abnormal, his father likens it to red currant jelly. He feels nauseated but has not vomited. On examination he has a palpable mass in his right lower quadrant but is not guarding and does not appear to be clinically peritonitic.

83 A 7-year-old boy presents to his GP with a new-onset abdominal pain in the past 24 hours. In addition he notes abdominal distension and constipation for the preceding 2 days. There is evidence of a right-sided abdominal mass which is resonant to percussion and he is afebrile with no other abdominal findings.

84 A 6-week-old infant is brought to see his GP as he is suffering from more frequent episodes of projectile vomiting. His mother is nervous as she has not had any other children and he appears to be hungry immediately after vomiting unaltered milk.

85 A 14-year-old girl is sent home from school after complaining of abdominal pain. She describes the pain as being increasingly constant in the right iliac fossa and has some associated diarrhoea and nausea. On examination she is found to be febrile and have tenderness in the right iliac fossa with some guarding.

Peri-arrest drugs

a. Atropine.

b. Adrenaline.

c. Amiodarone.

d. Lignocaine.

e. Magnesium sulphate.

f. Adenosine.

g. Verapamil.

h. Flecainide.

86 This is the drug of choice in sinus, artrial or nodal bradycardias.

It can also be used in pulseless electrical activity with a rate less than 60 beats per minute.

87 This drug is used in the management of torsades de pointes, ventricular tachyarrhythmias and occasionally in acute asthma.

88 Used in refractory ventricular fibrillation (VF) or pulseless ventricular tachycardia (VT).

89 Used in paroxysmal supraventricular tachycardia and narrow complex tachycardia.

90 Used in artrial fibrillation or supraventricular tachycardias with an accessory pathway.

Questions

Multiple choice questions (single best answer)

1 A 15-year-old boy is referred to the renal clinic by his GP with a history of worsening haematuria. His mother has been worried recently that he has been taking illicit drugs as he has been finding it more difficult to cope at school and has been falling behind in his schoolwork. He also seems to be less attentive of late and has become more withdrawn, watching tele vision on his own with the volume up loud. Which of the following conditions fits most closely with the clinical history?

☐ a. Alport's syndrome.

☐ b. Anderson–Fabry disease.

☐ c. Goodpasture's syndrome.

☐ d. Wegener's granulomatosis.

☐ e. Von Hippel–Lindau syndrome.

2 An 80-year-old woman presents to hospital with confusion and pain in her back. She was found by a neighbour wandering near her flat in the early hours of the evening stating that she was going to go to church. Routine blood tests in accident and emergency demonstrate a calcium of 3.1mmol/L, alkaline phosphatase of 249IU/L, urea of 12mmol/L with creatinine of 317mmol/L and a haemoglobin level of 10.7g/dL. Plain lumbosacral radiographs were done after eliciting point tenderness over the lower vertebrae that demonstrate punched-out lytic lesions. Which of the following is the most likely diagnosis?

☐ a. Paget's disease.

☐ b. Sarcoidosis.

☐ c. Hyperparathyroidism.

☐ d. Myeloma.

□ e. Osteosarcoma.

3 Which of the following is NOT routinely considered as part of a renal screen in the investigation of new-onset renal failure?

□ a. Complement.

□ b. Renal ultrasound.

□ c. Caeruloplasmin and serum copper.

□ d. Anti-neutrophil cytoplasmic antibodies.

□ e. Bence–Jones protein.

4 A 58-year-old woman presents to hospital with headache, blurred vision and palpitations. She states that she has been feeling unwell for about a week prior to coming to hospital and has been having more frequent headaches that are 'all over' her head and associated with blurring of her vision. Her past medical history is unremarkable. She tells you that she is worried that this might be a stroke as her two of her family members suffered from strokes at a young age. Routine observations record a blood pressure reading of 194/110mmHg with a pulse of 115 beats per minute, temperature of 36.4C with respiratory rate of 22 breaths per minute and oxygen saturations of 99% on room air. Examination findings are unremarkable. Routine blood tests show a sodium level of 136mmol/L, a potassium of 4.8mmol/L with a urea of 10.2mmol/L, creatinine of 172μmol/L and haemoglobin of 9.8g/dL. White cell count and C-reactive protein (CRP) are within normal limits.

Which of the following investigations in indicated in the first line?

□ a. Renal ultrasound.

□ b. CT scan of the head.

□ c. Renal biopsy.

□ d. 24-hour urinary metanephrines (VMA).

☐ e. Carotid and vertebral artery Dopplers.

5 A 5-year-old boy is referred to the paediatric nephrology clinic by his GP. His father states that his son has been passing dark urine that resembles blackcurrant juice and has noticed that his abdomen has become more swollen on one side than the other.

His father is worried that this might be cancer as his own mother died of breast cancer when he was 17 years old. On examination there is a painless mass that moves with respiration in the right flank and a urine sample performed at the clinic shows frank haematuria. Which of the following investigations is most important to obtain with respect to future management?

☐ a. CT scan of the abdomen.

☐ b. Renal ultrasonography.

☐ c. Bilateral surgical biopsies.

☐ d. Albumin/creatinine ratio.

☐ e. Chest radiography.

6 A 34-year-old man is brought to hospital short of breath and diagnosed with a chest infection. He is treated on amoxicillin and clarithromycin. Shortly after commencement of antibiotic therapy he is found on the ward to be passing only 10mL/h via his urinary catheter although he is well hydrated. Observations reveal a temperature of 38.4C, blood pressure of 165/96mmHg with a regular pulse of 92 beats per minute (bpm). Examination reveals a diffuse rash over his body. Urinalysis reveals proteinuria and eosinophils and blood tests reveal a markedly raised eosinophil count. Which of the following diagnoses is the most likely?

☐ a. Ascending urinary tract infection.

☐ b. Haemolytic uraemic syndrome.

☐ c. Drug-induced interstitial nephritis.

☐ d. Cholesterol embolus.

☐ e. Acute tubular necrosis.

7 Whilst on ward cover one evening you are asked to review a 78-year-old lady who is known to have a history of ischaemic heart disease and atrial fibrillation. She was admitted to hospital on this occasion after developing a severe community acquired pneumonia requiring intravenous treatment. The nursing staff are concerned that she seems to have developed a facial asymmetry which was not mentioned in her initial clerking. On your review she notes that this has been there for some time and her GP was investigating the cause prior to her admission into hospital. Which of the following is not known to cause a lower motor neurone facial weakness?

☐ a. Head injury.

☐ b. Sarcoidosis.

☐ c. Guillain–Barré syndrome.

☐ d. Lyme disease.

☐ e. Medullary infarction.

8 On your emergency medicine rotation you are clerking a 25-year-old patient who has presented with headaches. On the basis of the history you decide that these sound like tension headaches and neurological examination is perfectly normal apart from small pupils that you have noticed. They are equal and reactive to light and accommodation. In which of the following conditions are small pupils characteristic?

☐ a. Holmes–Adie syndrome.

☐ b. Acute retrobulbar neuritis.

☐ c. Amitriptyline overdose.

☐ d. Pontine haemorrhage.

☐ e. Syphilis.

9 During a busy medical take your Senior House Officer asks you to see a patient who has been referred by accident and emergency with a spastic

paraparesis. The patient is a 65-year-old gentleman who denies any past medical problems other than hypertension and an appendicectomy as a child. The family are concerned that this is due to the effect of a stroke and are concerned since he is a non-smoker and has no past cardiac problems. On examination you confirm that he does have a spastic paraparesis. Which of the following conditions would NOT be consistent with that clinical finding?

☐ a. Demyelating myelopathy.

☐ b. Spondylosis of the lumbosacral spine.

☐ c. Motor neurone disease.

☐ d. Syringomyelia.

☐ e. Meningioma.

10 Which of the following associations is incorrect?

☐ a. Hyponatraemia and central pontine myelinolysis.

☐ b. Hyperthyroidism and tremor.

☐ c. Hypernatraemia and seizures.

☐ d. Hypoglycaemia and hemiparesis.

☐ e. Hypercalcaemia and muscle cramps.

11 A 57-year-old gentleman presents to his GP having noticed that the power in his hand has reduced. He works as a carpen-ter and has noticed that he is finding it increasingly difficult to carry out tasks that he once considered effortless. He denies any weakness elsewhere and neurological examination is normal other than wasting and weakness in the hypothenar and small muscles of his right hand. Which of the following would NOT account for these signs?

☐ a. Peripheral motor neuropathies.

☐ b. Syringomyelia.

☐ c. Ulnar nerve lesion at the elbow.

☐ d. Amyotropic lateral sclerosis (ALS).

☐ e. Osteoarthritis of cervical and thoracic spine.

12 Whilst on your general practice rotation there is concern about a possible local outbreak of bovine spongiform encephalop athy.

During the following week you get a number of visits from patients concerned that this will develop into the human form of the disease and are concerned about the risks. Which of the following facts about Creutzfeld–Jakob disease are INCORRECT?

☐ a. It is caused by a slowly mutating virus.

☐ b. A typical presentation would involve a progressive dementia.

☐ c. It has been shown to be transmissible by surgery.

☐ d. Arises from a conformational change in a prion protein.

☐ e. Can be tested for with tonsil biopsies.

13 A 78-year-old man presents to hospital after not passing stool for 3 days. He is confused and is accompanied by his carer from the nursing home in which he is resident. A careful history from his daughter reveals he has lost 8 kg in weight over the past 2 months and has been acting unusually over the past month or so. Which of the following tumour markers would be expected to be raised in this disease?

a. Carcino-embryonic antigen (CEA).

b. CA 153.

c. Alpha-fetoprotein (AFP).

d. Neurone specific enolase (NSE).

e. Human chorionic gonadotrophin (HCG).

14 A 45-year-old woman is admitted electively to hospital for hepatic cyst fenestration. She makes a good post-operative recovery, however, on the 4th day post-surgery she starts to complain of abdominal pain with fever, nausea and a tender, tense abdomen. Routine blood tests show a high white cell count, a bilirubin of 32 µmol/L, alanine aminotransferase (ALT) of 50 µmol/L and an aspartate transaminase (AST) of 32 µmol/L.

Which of the following is the most sensitive diagnostic investigation to perform?

a. Ultra Sound liver and gallbladder.

b. HIDA scan.

c. Plain abdominal radiograph.

d. CT scan of the abdomen.

e. ERCP (endoscopic retrograde cholangiopancreatography).

15 A 67-year-old lady completed a week-long course of antibiotics for a hospital-acquired pneumonia. You are reviewing her and she complains that she feels generally unwell. Her observation chart shows a swinging fever and she notes that she is still suffering with a productive cough with foul-smelling sputum. On further questioning she admits chest pain and occasional haemoptysis. You request a chest X-ray and the results show a walled cavity. Which of the following is the most likely diagnosis?

☐ a. Pleural effusion.

☐ b. Pulmonary embolus.

☐ c. Recurrent infection.

☐ d. Lung abscess.

☐ e. Empyema.

16 Mr Davies is a 58-year-old gentleman with a history of recurrent pneumonia. He has been referred to the on-call team for management of this current episode of pneumonia as the GP is concerned that he is not able to get on top of this problem in the community. On further questioning you discover that he has been complaining of a persistent cough for the past 2 weeks with copious sputum that is occasionally bloodstained. He is a non-smoker. On examination you note finger clubbing with coarse inspiratory crepitations and occasional wheeze. An erect chest X-ray shows cystic shadows. Which of the following is the most likely diagnosis?

☐ a. Lung cancer.

☐ b. Bronchiectasis.

☐ c. Pulmonary fibrosis.

☐ d. Pneumonia.

☐ e. Pulmonary embolus.

17 You are asked to review a chest X-ray for a colleague. You notice a round opacity which of the following is NOT one of your differential diagnoses?

☐ a. Tuberculosis.

☐ b. Aspergilloma.

☐ c. Lung cancer.

☐ d. Sarcoidosis.

☐ e. Carcinoid tumour.

18 An 69-year-old gentleman with a past history of lung cancer presents with general fatigue and worsening shortness of breath.

He has been undergoing chemotherapy for his lung cancer and is due to be followed up with his oncologist in a few days time.

Which of the following are NOT known to be complications of lung cancer?

☐ a. Hyponatraemia.

☐ b. Superior vena cava obstruction.

☐ c. Hoarse voice.

☐ d. Horner's syndrome.

☐ e. Pulmonary oedema.

19 Causes of type I respiratory failure include all of the following except?

☐ a. Pneumonia.

☐ b. Pulmonary embolus.

☐ c. Acute exacerbation of asthma.

☐ d. Acute respiratory distress syndrome.

☐ e. Pulmonary fibrosis.

20 According to the British Thoracic Society, which of the following is NOT a major risk factor for a pulmonary embolus?

☐ a. Abdominal malignancy.

☐ b. Recent hip replacement.

☐ c. Oral contraceptive pill.

☐ d. Previous venous thromboembolism.

☐ e. Immobility.

21 Chest radiography confirms a pleural effusion and a pleural tap and drainage is performed. Pleural fluid analysis reveals a murky dark brown fluid with a protein content of 45g/dL and heavy lymphocytic involvement. Which of the following is the LEAST likely diagnosis?

☐ a. Tuberculosis.

☐ b. Malignancy.

☐ c. Rheumatoid arthritis.

☐ d. Liver failure.

☐ e. Systemic lupus erythematosus.

22 A 44-year-old man is brought in to accident and emergency by helicopter having fallen out of a third floor building. On arrival he has a Glasgow Coma Scale of 4/15 and is intubated and ventilated. Neurological examination reveals unequal pupils and urgent CT scan of the head is performed, which demonstrates midline shift and a left-sided convex enhancing area. Which of the following is the next most appropriate course of action?

☐ a. Intravenous mannitol to reduce intracranial pressure.

☐ b. Conservative management with 30 degree head-up nursing.

☐ c. Intravenous thiopentone to reduce intracranial pressure.

☐ d. Urgent neurosurgical evacuation of extradural haematoma.

☐ e. Urgent coiling of burst aneurysm under neuroradiological guidance.

23 A 47-year-old business man is caught in a fire in his office and suffers severe burns to his arms and upper body. He is assessed to have 35% burns to the upper torso, which are not painful to touch and are white in colour. He is admitted to hospital and placed under observation in the burns unit. Which of the following complications of this type of injury is especially important to recognise?

☐ a. Respiratory distress.

☐ b. Bacterial infection.

☐ c. Loss of peripheral pulses.

☐ d. Severe dehydration.

☐ e. Acute stress ulceration.

24 An adolescent presents to his school doctor with bilateral tender and swollen breasts. He has become increasingly self-conscious of late and has been avoiding physical education classes. On examination there are tender soft masses in the lower quadrants of both breasts. Which of the following is the most appropriate next step in managing this patient?

☐ a. Urgent referral to social services.

□ b. Reassure the patient that this is normal.

□ c. Needle aspiration and send fluid for culture and cytology.

□ d. Referral to a breast surgeon for excision and biopsy.

□ e. Short course of oral prednisolone and 2-week review.

25 A 43-year-old man comes to hospital with severe pain and tenderness in the left flank. A provisional diagnosis of ureteric obstruction by a renal calculus is made. Intravenous urogram taken shortly after admission to hospital would be most likely to show:

□ a. Reduced size of left kidney.

□ b. Reduced size of right kidney.

□ c. Perfusion defect in the left pelvicalyxceal region.

□ d. Bladder residual post-micturition.

□ e. Delayed excretion by left kidney.

26 A 31-year-old woman is admitted to the surgical team with nausea, bilious vomiting and generalised abdominal pain. She has had multiple previous admissions for abdominal pain and bloody diarrhoea and takes regular low-dose steroids under review by the gastroenterologists. Abdominal X-ray performed on admission demonstrates dilated loops of small bowel. Which of the following is the most likely cause of the radiological findings?

☐ a. Meckel's diverticulum.

☐ b. Intussusception.

☐ c. Adhesions.

☐ d. Stricture due to ulcerative colitis.

☐ e. Gastro-colic fistula due to Crohn's disease.

27 A 12-year-old boy presents to his GP with several days of generalised tiredness, painful joints in particular the knees, nodular swelling over his elbows and associated low-grade fever with a mild rash on his chest. He has no other medical problems but a few weeks earlier he had complained of a sore throat, which was managed supportively. Which of the following is the most likely diagnosis?

☐ a. Rheumatic fever.

☐ b. Rheumatoid arthritis.

☐ c. Reiter's syndrome.

☐ d. Scarlet fever.

☐ e. Systemic lupus erythematosus.

91

28 A 5-year-old boy is brought to see this GP by his parents. He has never visited the practice before but his parents tell you that he has no past medical history of note. At present, they are concerned that he seems to tire easily and complain of pain in his legs. He prefers to stay indoor and watch television rather than playing outdoors with other children. On physical examination, he looks well. His blood pressure reads 138/94 mmHg in his right arm and his legs appear to be atrophic and mottled in colour. Which of the following findings are UNLIKELY to be present in this boy?

☐ a. Reduced lower extremity pulses.

☐ b. Cyanosis of the toes.

☐ c. A bicuspid aortic valve on echocardiography.

☐ d. Rib notching on chest X-ray.

☐ e. Left ventricular hypertrophy on ECG.

29 A 17-year-old girl seeks advice from her GP for severe abdominal pain. The pain started in her lower abdomen and is central.

She has some associated nausea but no vomiting. On further questioning she denies any disturbance to her bowels but notes some dyspareunia and admits to having had unprotected sexual intercourse. She has a low-grade fever and confirms a small amount of smelly vaginal discharge. Which of the following is the most likely diagnosis in this case?

☐ a. Endometriosis.

☐ b. Ruptured ovarian cyst.

☐ c. Pelvic inflammatory disease.

☐ d. Uterine fibroids.

☐ e. Mittelschmerz pain.

30 Which of the following facts about carcinoma of the cervix are INCORRECT?

☐ a. 90% are adenocarcinoma.

☐ b. Associated with human papilloma virus.

☐ c. Common presentation is intermenstrual vaginal bleeding.

☐ d. Cervical erosions may be seen on speculum examination.

☐ e. The disease may not present until the advanced stage.

31 A research fellow is assessing the effectiveness of a new surgical therapy for melanoma and recruits newly diagnosed melanoma sufferers to the study. He randomises the total participants to either the existing treatment or the novel treatment arm and performs the standard operation for melanoma excision on the first group (n 420). He also performs the newly proposed therapy on the second group (n 390). The treatment arms are double-blinded (both to him and the patients); 6 months after the surgery the patients are seen in clinic to assess for recurrence rates. The following data are obtained:

Disease present

Disease absent

Standard treatment

80

340

Novel treatment

60

330

Which of the following investigations would be the most suitable for investigating the effect of the novel treatment?

☐ a. Mann–Whitney U test

☐ b. Paired t-test

☐ c. Positive-predictive value

94

□ d. Odds ratio

□ e. Chi-squared test

32 A 37-year-old lady was admitted to hospital at 2 a.m. following a fall out of her first floor bedroom window. The incidents surrounding the accident were unclear but on arrival to hospital she was immobilised in a hard collar and sandbags and had a GCS of 15 with an obvious left-sided distal radial fracture. On further examination she was found to have left-sided bony pelvic pain which on X-ray was found to be a fracture of the iliac wing. She denied any pain in her thoracic and lumbar spine during a log roll examination and the rectal examination was found to be unremarkable. Examination of her cervical spine elicited no bony tenderness and good flexion and extension without development of any paraesthesiae or pain. Antero-posterior, lateral and peg views of her cervical spine showed no evidence of any fractures, subluxations or dislocations. How should we proceed from here?

□ a. Remove hard collar and three-way immobilisation.

□ b. Keep just hard collar on.

□ c. Keep hard collar and three-way immobilisation in situ and organise CT of the cervical spine to confirm the X-ray findings.

□ d. Remove hard collar but organise CT of cervical spine urgently

□ e. Get flexion and extension cervical spine views.

95

33 Which of the following signs is NOT an early sign of compartment syndrome?

☐ a. Pain in the affected limb on passive movements.

☐ b. Pallor.

☐ c. Tension of the muscle group.

☐ d. Loss of pulse.

☐ e. Paraesthesiae.

34 An 87-year-old man is admitted to hospital for shortness of breath and coughing up bloodstained sputum. A chest radiograph demonstrates a ring-shadow in the right upper lobe and CT scan of the chest is suspicious for malignancy. Bronchoscopy and histology confirms the diagnosis. The family are involved daily in the care of the patient and one day the daughters

approach you and urge you that if the diagnosis is cancer then for the sake of their father's state of mind can you tell him the results are inconclusive. The family tell you they have just bur-ied their mother having died of breast cancer and they fear their father will not be able to take the news. Which of the following is the correct course of action?

☐ a. Comply with their wishes to not let their father know the diagnosis on grounds of compassion.

☐ b. Only disclose the diagnosis to the father if he asks directly.

☐ c. Allow the grieving period to come to a close and let his GP break the diagnosis once out of hospital.

☐ d. State that you understand the delicate situation but inform the patient of his diagnosis as it is his right to know.

☐ e. Ask the family to break the diagnosis to their father at an appropriate time.

35 A 54-year-old man presents with pain in his left knee and a rash on his forearm that he has noticed developing over some weeks. He describes the rash as red underneath with a white

scale that can be rubbed off to leave little spots of bleeding. The rash is confined to the forearm and involves the elbow and there is a little area of similar looking rash over an old appendix scar. He has also noticed some differences in two of the nails of his right hand with little roughened depressions in the nails themselves. He is seen by his GP who diagnoses the condition and prescribes some medication. Which of the following is NOT used in the treatment of the above skin disorder?

☐ a. Topical steroids.

☐ b. Tar.

☐ c. Aqueous cream.

☐ d. PUVA.

☐ e. Dapsone.

36 A 6-year-old girl is brought to her GP by her mother who has noticed that she has been scratching incessantly and has become extremely irritable over the past week. The mother can identify no precipitants, however, states that the girl has recently started at a new school and asks if it could be something to do with this. On examination there is a widespread rash over the abdomen with tiny papules over the webspaces and fingers of both hands that are intensely itchy. Associated with the papules are linear tracts that are surrounded by erythema. Which of the following treatments should be instituted?

☐ a. Malathion 0.5% cream.

☐ b. Flucloxacillin 500mg.

☐ c. Conservative management.

☐ d. Topical aqueous cream.

☐ e. Cold tar.

37 A 73-year-old lady presents to the on-call surgical team complaining of right-sided abdominal pain. On further questioning the pain is mainly in the right flank but does radiate down to the groin. She has noticed dysuria and associated nausea, fever and rigors. On examination there are no palpable masses but she has tenderness on palpation of the renal angle. Urine dipstick is

positive for leucocytes, nitrites, glucose and blood.

Observations include a temperature of 38.0°C, RR 24/min, Sats 87%, HR 92/min and BP 109/64 mmHg. Which of the following is the most appropriate management for this patient?

☐ a. Oral antibiotics and community follow-up.

☐ b. i.v. antibiotics and i.v. fluids.

☐ c. Catheterise.

☐ d. Analgesia.

☐ e. Diuretics and i.v. fluids.

38 A 71-year-old man is admitted semi-electively for an anterior resection for a sigmoid cancer. Initial appearances on colonoscopy and CT scanning suggest that the cancer is confined to the bowel. He has been admitted a couple of days early since he is now obstipated and suffering colicky central abdominal pains.

The colicky pain is now becoming more constant and there is some concern that he is becoming obstructed. In addition, he notes some dysuria and difficulty in passing urine. What is the likely cause for his urinary symptoms?

☐ a. Prostatic metastases.

☐ b. Pyelonephritis.

☐ c. Bladder cancer.

☐ d. External pressure on urinary system.

☐ e. Urinary tract infection.

39 A 67-year-old woman presents to accident and emergency with right-sided chest pain and some shortness of breath. Examination reveals a pleural effusion which is confirmed on chest X-ray.

Aspiration of the fluid identifies less than 30g of protein. Which of the following would not be consistent with the above picture?

☐ a. Hypothyroidism.

☐ b. Liver cirrhosis.

☐ c. Nephrotic syndrome.

☐ d. Pneumonia.

☐ e. Cardiac failure.

40 A university health care centre doctor is called to see a student who

100

has been unwell by worried friends. He has not been attending lectures of late and has been feeling feverish and hot for the last 24 hours. There is an empty packet of ibuprofen 400mg by his bedside and it is decided to start benzylpenicillin empirically to cover for meningitis. As he is transferred to hospital the ambulance crew notice a non-blanching rash over his right thigh. In hospital his temperature is recorded at 39.1°C and he has started to vomit. Blood cultures are sent off on admission to hospital. What is the most likely cause of vomiting in this man?

☐ a. Idiosyncratic reaction to ibuprofen.

☐ b. Allergic reaction to benzylpenicillin.

☐ c. Neurogenic (central) reaction.

☐ d. Systemic inflammatory response to infection.

☐ e. NSAID irritation to gastric mucosa.

41 A 63-year-old gentleman was admitted to hospital after suffering with a transient ischaemic attack (TIA). He noticed weakness in his right arm and some changes in his speech, both of which were completely resolved in the 24 hours after onset.

On examination, he had no residual neurological findings and no cardiovascular findings of note. Which investigations would be useful to determine the cause for this event and likelihood of future episodes?

☐ a. MRI brain.

□ b. Chest X-ray.

□ c. Abdominal ultrasound scan.

□ d. Carotid Doppler scanning.

□ e. ECG.

42 A 63-year-old man is brought to hospital by ambulance following a fall at home. He lives alone and is unaccompanied to hospital. On arrival he is assessed by the emergency staff and appears confused and disorientated but moving all four limbs and communicating, albeit inappropriately. His urine dipstick is positive for leucocytes, nitrites and protein. He scores 3/10 on the abbreviated mental test (AMT) and is uncooperative with physical examination, pulling out his intravenous lines and trying to leave the hospital. Which of the following medications would be of most benefit in managing this patient?

□ a. Haloperidol.

□ b. Lorazepam.

□ c. Memantine.

□ d. Olanzipine.

□ e. Sertraline.

43 A 43-year-old woman is brought to hospital by her husband after he found she had taken an overdose of her medication in her bathroom. Her past medical history is remarkable for hypertension and depression. She denies taking any medication overdose, stating that her husband is simply worrying unnecessarily.

On examination she is drowsy with dilated pupils and sluggish reflexes. A tachycardia is clinically evident and electrocardiography is performed that demonstrates a prolonged PR and

QT interval. Which of the following medications is most likely responsible for her symptoms?

☐ a. Tranylcypromine.

☐ b. Amitriptyline.

☐ c. Digoxin.

☐ d. Atenolol.

☐ e. Sertraline.

44 A 25-year-old man presents to his GP complaining of difficulty sleeping. He complains that he feels very hot at night and finds that his work is suffering during the day. Otherwise he complains of no problems, but on questioning he admits to slight weight loss and examination reveals a unilateral cervical mass.

The mass is in the anterior compartment of the neck; it is not tethered to the skin and does not move on swallowing or protrusion of the tongue. What is the most likely diagnosis in this case?

☐ a. Hodgkin's lymphoma.

☐ b. Sarcoidosis.

☐ c. Tuberculosis.

☐ d. Anxiety.

☐ e. Acute lymphocytic leukaemia.

45 A 70-year-old lady presents to her GP with vague aches and pains particularly in her back. Other symptoms include polyuria and constipation. She has noticed that she is more prone to picking chest infections over the past few months. An X-ray shows two crush fractures of her lumbar vertebrae. Blood tests taken show a calcium level of 2.96 with a normal albumin level and Phosphate level 0.9. What is the likely diagnosis?

☐ a. Myeloma.

☐ b. Myelofibrosis.

☐ c. Myelodysplasia.

☐ d. Adrenal tumour.

☐ e. Prolapsed lumbar disc.

46 A 45-year-old woman presents to accident and emergency with abdominal pain. She is tested for pregnancy, urinary tract infection and undergoes abdominal examination. She is found to have an enlarged spleen with pain localised to the left upper quadrant. Blood tests reveal a haemoglobin level of 9.8 g/dL

with an mean cell volume (MCV) of 92 fL. WBC was 26 109 and platelet count was 135 109. Which of the following chromosomal translocations is most likely to be found in sufferers of this condition?

☐ a. t(8;14)

☐ b. t(9;22)

☐ c. t(14;21)

☐ d. t(11;22)

☐ e. t(4;14)

47 Which of the following modalities represents the most useful indicator of the severity of disease in a rheumatoid arthritis sufferer?

☐ a. Serial radiographs of hands and wrists.

☐ b. Commencement of biological agents.

☐ c. Ability to dress and care for oneself.

☐ d. Number of visits to hospital.

☐ e. Length of treatment with steroids.

48 A 32-year-old woman presents to hospital with weakness in her left leg and arm with an obvious facial droop on the left hand side. History taking reveals a sudden onset of loss of function of the left side of her body with no loss of consciousness, tongue-biting or associated incontinence of faeces or urine. Past medical history is remarkable only for four miscarriages and peptic ulcer disease. Which of the following diagnoses is most likely?

☐ a. Systemic sclerosis.

☐ b. Marfan's syndrome.

☐ c. Dermatomyositis.

☐ d. Antiphospholipid syndrome.

☐ e. Reiter's syndrome.

106

49 A 23-year-old girl is referred to the breast clinic by her GP. She first sought advice when she noticed a solitary lump in the upper outer aspect of her left breast. She notes that the lump is not painful and there are no overlying changes to the skin. She has no history of breast problems and has no family history of breast cancer. There has been no change in the size of the lump and no association with her menstrual cycle. She admits that it has been present for more than a month but she was too nervous to have it investigated. She denies using any regular medications. Which of the following is the most likely diagnosis?

☐ a. Fibroadenoma.

☐ b. Ductal carcinoma in situ.

☐ c. Invasive ductal carcinoma.

☐ d. Breast cyst.

☐ e. Breast abscess.

50 A 69-year-old gentleman is seen by his GP for gradual onset gynaecomastia. The patient has tolerated the development of the condition hoping that it would resolve spontaneously

although it continues to gradually worsen. He has a history of alcohol abuse, drinking approximately 70 units per week and has been hospitalised with pancreatitis and acute liver failure in the past. Which of the following is the most likely cause for his gynaecomastia?

☐ a. Physiological.

☐ b. Liver failure.

☐ c. Kleinfelter's syndrome.

☐ d. Hyperthyroidism.

☐ e. Drugs including spironolactone.

51 A 74-year-old woman is referred to accident and emergency with a history of pain and redness in her right eye that is associated with blurred vision and distortion of her vision leading her to see 'haloes' around objects. When asked if anything makes the pain better or worse she tells you that it seems to come on in the early evening. Which of the following diagnoses is the most likely?

☐ a. Endophthalmitis.

☐ b. Acute glaucoma.

☐ c. Retinitis pigmentosa.

☐ d. Retinal detachment.

☐ e. Retinal artery occlusion.

52 A 59-year-old man presents to hospital with progressive deterioration in visual acuity over as period of weeks such that he had trouble focussing on even the closest of objects and had had to stop driving completely. He found that he was experiencing glare when in bright sunlight and had taken to wearing sun-glasses when outside. On examination there was frank opacity of the left pupil with reduced clarity of the right pupil and visual acuity was reduced to hand waving in the left eye. Which of the following has NOT been associated with the development of posterior subcapsular cataract?

☐ a. Obesity.

☐ b. Steroids.

☐ c. Hypertriglyceridaemia.

☐ d. Hypertension.

☐ e. Hypoglycaemia.

53 A 72-year-old woman presents to hospital with shortness of breath. She is found to have a significant cardiac history of ischaemic heart disease with previous coronary artery bypass grafting and ventricular arrhythmias, which she has had for many years. As part of the work-up for shortness of breath she has blood tests taken that demonstrate a slightly high white cell count and C-reactive protein. Thyroid function test, however, returns abnormal. Which of the following medications is most likely responsible for the deterioration in thyroid function?

□ a. Atenolol.

□ b. Atorvastatin.

□ c. Amlodipine.

□ d. Amiodarone.

□ e. Acarbose.

54 Regarding hyperthyroidism, which of the following statements is correct?

□ a. T3 is more abundantly produced than T4.

□ b. Lid retraction can be used to monitor therapy.

□ c. Beta-blockade is always required long term for tachycardia.

□ d. T4 is more potent than T3.

□ e. High T4, T3 and TSH levels are seen in thyrotoxicosis.

55 A 75-year-old gentleman is admitted to hospital following intermittent chest pain for the past 24 hours. His chest pain was central in location with no radiation but was relieved by GTN spray in 3 minutes. His troponin level was positive and ECG showed fixed inverted T waves laterally. He has a past history of peripheral vascular disease. The next stage of his management should include:

☐ a. An exercise tolerance test (ETT).

☐ b. A thallium cardiac scan.

☐ c. Serial ECGs.

☐ d. CT chest.

☐ e. Coronary angiogram.

56 A 78-year-old lady was referred to the cardiologist during her inpatient stay for increasing attacks of angina. She is currently using PRN GTN spray, verapamil and enalapril. She has noticed that the frequency of her angina attacks is increasing and her symptoms are becoming more severe at rest. What changes in her medications will improve her symptoms?

☐ a. Change verapamil to diltiazem and start isosorbide mononitrate.

☐ b. Give regular nitrates.

111

☐ c. Change ace inhibitor.

☐ d. Add in beta-blocker.

☐ e. Start digoxin.

57 An 81-year-old gentleman is admitted to hospital with chest pain and a diagnosis of a Non-ST Elevation MI (NSTEMI) is made.

Which of the following is the most appropriate immediate medical management?

☐ a. Aspirin, warfarin and beta-blocker.

☐ b. Aspirin, clopidogrel, clexane and GTN spray.

☐ c. Clopidogrel, GTN spray and warfarin.

☐ d. Clopidogrel, clexane and warfarin.

☐ e. Clexane, warfarin, beta-blocker and statin.

58 A 58-year-old man presents with new-onset chest pain and shortness of breath. ECG shows atrial fibrillation with a rate of 180 beats per minute. He has no past cardiac history. The most appropriate management would be:

☐ a. Oxygen, digoxin i.v.

☐ b. Oxygen, beta-blockers.

☐ c. Oxygen, heparin, warfarin.

☐ d. Oxygen, heparin, i.v. amiodarone.

☐ e. Oxygen, heparin and synchronized DC shock.

59 A 70-year-old man presents with chest pain. His ECG shows an acute myocardial infraction (MI) with a new left bundle branch block. On admission he is given 100% oxygen, morphine, meto-clopramide, GTN spray and aspirin. On further questioning you elicit that he suffered a haemorrhagic stroke a year ago. The next most appropriate step in management is:

☐ a. Coronary artery bypass surgery.

☐ b. Thrombolytic therapy with streptokinase.

☐ c. Percutaneous transluminal coronary angioplasty (PTCA).

☐ d. Heparin infusion.

☐ e. i.v. glycoprotein lib/IIIa inhibitor.

60 Which of the following is NOT a contraindication to thrombolysis following a diagnosis of an acute MI?

☐ a. Previous allergic reaction.

☐ b. Cerebral infarct 2 years ago.

☐ c. Suspected aortic dissection.

☐ d. Heavy vaginal bleeding.

☐ e. Hypotension.

Extended matching questions

Glomerulonephritides

a. Minimal change disease.

b. IgA nephropathy (Berger's disease).

c. Focal segmental glomerulosclerosis.

d. Post-streptococcal glomerulonephritis.

e. Rapidly progressive glomerulonephritis (RPGN).

f. Membranous glomerulonephritis.

g. Wegener's granulomatosis.

h. Henoch–Schönlein purpura (HSP).

i. Systemic-lupus erythematosus.

The following patients have all presented with renal disease. Please choose the most likely option from the list above. Each option can be used once, more than once or not at all.

61 A 10-year-old boy is brought to hospital with a rash over his buttocks associated with abdominal pain and vomiting. In accident and emergency he is accompanied by his mother and

stepfather. His mother had left him for the weekend with the stepfather and was called to come back from her holiday as he had started to have some bloody stools associated with the rash. Social services had been notified on arrival to hospital.

62 A 30-year-old man presents to hospital complaining that his urine has been very dark recently, resembling coffee at worst.

He has been under the weather recently and has taken a few days off work with a very sore throat and coryzal symptoms.

Urine dipstick in hospital returns highly positive for blood and protein. He is admitted for supportive management and is scheduled for a renal biopsy, which shows mesangial proliferation with a positive immunofluorescence pattern.

63 A 5-year-old boy is referred to hospital and seen with his father who is worried that he has been listless. He is not sure why his GP suggested he should come to accident and emergency and is keen to 'get some tablets and go home'. On examination the child is tired and irritable and has some swelling around his eyes. Carefully considered renal biopsy is remarkable only for some podocyte fusion on electron microscopy.

64 A 40-year-old woman is admitted from accident and emergency

☐ with a history of arthralgia, facial rash, chest pain and neuropsychiatric symptoms. She is investigated for the cause of her symptoms and undergoes urine dipstick, simple blood tests, electrocardiology, porphyria and sickle screens and troponin initially. She is found to have renal failure with poor urine output and a decision to perform a renal biopsy is taken, which demonstrates wire-loop lesions on light microscopy

.

65 A 28-year-old man presents with shortness of breath, haemoptysis, swollen legs and face, and haematuria. He describes feeling progressively more unwell in the weeks preceding admission but was afraid that this 'might be the end'. Clinically he exhibits signs of renal failure and his blood results show a glomerular filtration rate of 8mL/min (severe). He is admitted to hospital and rapidly deteriorates over a matter of weeks requiring emergency renal replacement therapy. Autoantibody screen returns positive for anti-glomerular basement membrane and renal biopsy demonstrates a florid necrotising glomerulonephritis with crescent formation.

116

Dementia

a. Alzheimer's dementia.

b. Creutzfeldt–Jakob disease.

c. Multi-infarct dementia.

d. Frontotemporal dementia.

e. HIV dementia.

f. Alcohol-related dementia.

g. Lewy-body dementia.

h. Pseudo-dementia.

The following patients have all presented with dementia. Please choose the most correct diagnosis from the above list. Each option may be used once, more than once or not at all.

66 A 65-year-old man is brought to his GP by his wife. She is worried that recently he has been behaving more and more unusually and out of character for him. He has become more

forgetful of late and she often gets the impression that he has trouble focusing on her when she is talking to him. His past medical history details two previous admissions to hospital under the neurologists for transient ischaemic attack and stroke.

67 A 68-year-old man is brought to accident and emergency having fallen and broken his hip. Further questioning reveals he is confused and upon talking to a relative a history of tremors and long-standing hypertension is gained. Mini-mental state examination yields a score of 21 and on examination he exhibits bradykinesia, a shuffling gait and a unilateral tremor of his right hand. The relative states that he often seems to hal-lucinate and become restless.

68 A 61-year-old woman is brought in by the police to hospital found wandering at night in her dressing gown. Mini-mental state examination reveals a score of 18. Her daughter describes her mother as more aggressive recently and often has trouble remembering who she is when she comes to visit. The daughter also states that she has been told by her mother's neighbour on more than one occasion that he has been called at odd times in the night by her.

69 A 58-year-old woman, recently widowed, is brought to hospital by her relatives. She was found at home to have no food in her cupboard and a neighbour who helps her clean found her lying in bed in a poor state of hygiene. Her mini-mental state examination score was 24 and during the test she became very agitated and tearful.

70 A 31-year-old man from Botswana is brought to accident and emergency by the police. He was found at 2 o'clock in the morning holding a knife and wandering the street outside his house. He maintains that somebody is poisoning him and making him feel terrible and he complains of a 'flu-like illness'. On examination he is a slim man with poor nutrition and vital signs reveal a low-grade pyrexia.

Lower gastrointestinal bleeding

a. Angiodysplasia.

b. Osler–Weber–Rendu syndrome.

c. Colorectal carcinoma.

d. Haemorrhoids.

e. Drug-induced bleeding.

f. Mesenteric embolus.

g. Inflammatory bowel disease.

h. Diverticulitis.

i. Inherited coagulopathy.

j. Rectal polyp.

The following patients have all suffered from bleeding from the lower gastrointestinal tract. Please choose the more correct diagnosis from the above list. Each option may be used once, more than once or not at all.

71 A 43-year-old man presents with bright red rectal bleeding. He denies any pain and states that it came on suddenly with no warning. He has not had any change in bowel habit and does not take any regular medication. Past medical history is remarkable for a total knee replacement 5 years ago and an inpatient admission under the ENT surgeons for a severe nosebleed as a child.

72 A 62-year-old woman presents with rectal bleeding on passing stool. Bleeding is seen on the toilet paper and in the toilet bowl.

She states that she has had a few episodes of small fresh bleeding but denies any weight loss or diarrhoea. She describes a feeling of something descending in the rectum when she strains at stool and often feels the urge to defaecate but without success. In fact she suffers from constipation and is due to see her GP for a repeat prescription for senna and lactulose as she has run out.

73 A 67-year-old man presents with rectal bleeding with no warning or associated change in bowel habit. He has experienced episodes of bleeding like this in the past, which usually settle on their own. Referred by his GP to hospital for the last serious episode of rectal bleeding he underwent colonoscopy, which demonstrated a small vascular abnormality.

74 A 54-year-old man presents to the dermatology clinic with a history of multiple red lesions on his nose and around his mouth. He has been suffering recurrent nosebleeds intermittently since he was a child and has had the lesions as long as he can remember. Past medical history is remarkable only for an aspirin allergy that caused severe rectal bleeding. On examination there are multiple, small red lesions that blanch on pressure over them distributed over the face, lips, nose and mouth.

75 A 67-year-old man complains of abdominal pain and rectal bleeding. He has recently been started on digoxin and atenolol for an episode of shortness of breath and palpitations and was due for an anticoagulation clinic appointment to commence on warfarin. He is brought to hospital collapsed in the street and had passed fresh blood per rectum in accident and emergency.

Clinically he exhibits signs of shock and requires fluid resuscitation and blood transfusion.

Shortness of breath

a. Atelectasis.

b. Lung cancer.

c. Aspiration pneumonia.

d. Pneumothorax.

e. Exacerbation of asthma/COPD.

f. Pulmonary embolus.

g. Congestive cardiac failure.

76 A 74-year-old gentleman is 1 day post-operatively from his total hip replacement for the treatment of arthritis affecting his hip.

Immediately post-operatively he made a good recovery and did not complain of excessive pain. He has a history of COPD and hypertension but no other medical problems. The nurses are concerned about him as they have just done his observations and he has a temperature of 38.5°C, whilst he is not complaining of any pain he feels short of breath and has noticed a dry cough. What is the most likely cause for his shortness of breath?

77 You are a member of the cardiac arrest team and you are called to a medical ward where a patient has arrested. You remember the patient as you had been asked to see him previously to dose his warfarin as he was being treated for a pulmonary embolus. The nurses mention that he was complaining of increasing shortness of breath in the hours up to the arrest which seemed to be somewhat alleviated by administration of oxygen and his nebuliser. Upon attaching the cardiac monitor you note that the rhythm is asystole, despite 3 cycles of cardio-pulmonary resuscitation there is no change in his status and death is confirmed.

What is the likely cause for this man's demise?

78 An 80-year-old gentleman has been admitted for the investigation of his recurrent falls. A full screen of blood tests including a full blood count and urea and electrolytes has shown no abnormalities. You come to review him after the weekend on Monday morning and the nursing staff are concerned that he is not quite himself. He appears to be slumped over to one side and you notice some slurred speech. You are told by the nursing staff that he has been eating well over the weekend but they have noticed that he has developed a cough this morning.What is the most likely diagnosis in this case?

79 A 49-year-old lady presents with increasing shortness of breath.She was seen by her GP earlier in the day who was concerned that clinically she had a pleural effusion and asked her to attend accident and emergency for an urgent chest X-ray and medical review. She is normally fit and well and works as a banker. Of late she has been complaining of mild shortness of breath but she has attributed it to the fact that she has been smoking more than usual due to the stress of work. On clinical examination there are no peripheral signs of respiratory disease although her respiratory rate is 20/min. There is dullness to percussion at the right base and reduced chest expansion and breath sounds in the same area. A chest X-ray confirms a pleural effusion, what is the likely

diagnosis?

80 A 74-year-old lady presents acutely short of breath. She mentions that she has been increasingly dyspnoeic over the past week but her breathing has worsened significantly over

the past 24 hours. She denies any associated chest pain but confirms that she has a slightly productive cough. On further questioning she admits that she could not pick up her repeat prescription for her inhalers as she was too short of breath and has been without her salbutamol and spiriva for 5 days. On examination her respiratory rate is 18/min and auscultation

reveals widespread wheeze with some crepitations heard in the left upper zone. What is the likely diagnosis?

Acute abdomen

a. Appendicitis.

b. Pancreatitis.

c. Diverticulitis.

d. Intussusception.

e. Sigmoid volvulus.

f. Perforated peptic ulcer.

123

g. Ruptured abdominal aortic aneurysm.

h. Basal pneumonia.

i. Rectosigmoid carcinoma.

j. Appendiceal carcinoid.

The following patients have all presented with abdominal complaints. Please choose the most correct diagnosis from the above list. Each option may be used once, more than once, or not at all.

81 A 15-year-old boy presents to his GP with a 2 day history of vomiting, nausea and loss of appetite. On examination he is generally tender but more so over the right side of his abdomen. Blood tests reveal a low-grade pyrexia, high white cell count and raised C-reactive protein.

82 A 65-year-old woman is brought to hospital complaining of bright red blood in her stools. On examination she is tender in the left iliac fossa with a hard non-fluctuant mass palpable in the same region. Blood tests reveal a high white cell count, C-reactive protein of 135 and a temperature of 37.9°C.

83 A 72-year-old man presents to accident and emergency with a history of weight loss, confusion and abdominal pain. He is from a nursing home where the nurses state that he has not opened his bowels for 2 days and has become increasingly unwell over the past few weeks. Blood results reveal a haemoglobin of 7.2 g/dL, MCV of 74.3 fL, urea of 9.4 mmol/L and creatinine of 155 mol/L.

84 A 45-year-old stockbroker presents to hospital complaining of severe abdominal pain. He states that he has not been eating for the past week due to pain and has felt nauseated and has vomited twice this morning. On examination his abdomen is tense with absent bowel sounds and is very tender over the epigastrium.

85 A 57-year-old woman is brought to hospital by ambulance with abdominal pain. She has vomited green fluid this morning and has been very constipated since yesterday. Past medical history reveals high blood pressure and cholesterol treated with atenolol and simvastatin. On examination she is sitting forward on the bed and in pain. Clinically the abdomen is exquisitely tender over the epigastrium. Bowel sounds are present and there are no masses. Chest examination reveals a respiratory rate of 26 breaths per minute with reduced breath sounds in the left base.

Relevant milestones

a. 0–3 months.

b. 3–6 months.

c. 6–9 months.

d. 9–12 months.

e. 12–18 months.

f. 18–24 months.

g. 2–5 years.

h. 5–10 years.

86 This child has a heart rate of 95–140/min, a respiratory rate of 25 breaths per minute, and a systolic BP of 90mmHg.

87 The child sits unaided.

88 First dose of diphtheria, tetanus, pertussis, polio, Haemophilus

☐ influenza B and meningitis C vaccination is administered in

accordance with the normal vaccination schedule in the United Kingdom.

89 Persistent runny nose, mild fever, shortness of breath with asso-

☐ ciated dry cough and wheeze. On examination accessory muscles are being used and there are fine end inspiratory crackles on the chest.

90 Able to follow movements with eyes.

☐

ANSWERS

Answers and notes

PAPER 1 ANSWERS

Multiple choice questions (single best answer)

1 d. An echocardiogram is the most important next step in the management of this gentleman. This will aid in the decision about anticoagulation. If an echocardiogram shows a structurally abnormal heart then the risk of thrombus formation is small and warfarinisation would be unnecessary. Whilst AF can commonly be managed in the community, it is appropriate to refer for ECHO. Rate control is unnecessary in this scenario as its upper limit is 90 beats per minute.

2 d. This gentleman can be safely discharged without follow-up.

The troponin results represent a 12-hour test by which time if there was cardiac damage the levels would have peaked. This combined with the fact that there are no ischaemic changes on the ECG make the risk of a cardiac event minimal. Having ruled out a cardiac cause for his chest pain a gastrointestinal cause is most likely given the associated nausea. There is no indication to start this gentleman on aspirin.

3 e. Measuring digoxin levels in this lady will detect any potential toxicity which would account for her symptoms. This case actually showed digoxin toxicity and a binding agent was administered. There is no indication to insert a pacing wire in this lady as her heart rate is being maintained at 40 beats per minute although there is complete heart block. Having stopped this lady's digoxin, her heart rate increased to approximately 120 beats per minute and ultimately she had a permanent pacemaker inserted.

Amiodarone is indicated in refractory tachycardias.

4 a. Ventricular septal rupture is a rare but serious complication of myocardial infarction. The event occurs 2–8 days after an infarction and often precipitates cardiogenic shock. Dressler's syndrome is a pericarditis that develops between 2 and 10 weeks post myocardial infarction or cardiac surgery. One theory is that it is an inflammatory response secondary to an autoimmune reaction to myocardial neoantigens.

5 a. This lady had no history of alcoholism and no signs of outflow tract obstruction. The most likely cause of her dilated cardiomyopathy is viral. The commonest viruses implicated in this condition are coxsackie A and B, influenza A and B adeno-virus and echovirus among others.

6 d. Whilst measuring the blood pressure in all limbs raises the suspicion of aortic dissection, the most diagnostic investigation is a CT chest. Other diagnostic investigations include MRI and a transoesophageal echocardiogram. There are no diagnostic ECG changes associated with dissecting aortic aneurysms and liver function tests are of no use in confirming the diagnosis.

7 c. This clinical picture is typical of diabetic ketoacidosis (DKA) occurring secondarily to a preceding infection. In times of stress, such as post-operatively, in the case of infection or inflammation or after an event such as a myocardial infarction, blood glucose levels may rise due to an increase in the stress response and release of gluconeogenic hormones. Insulin requirements may increase remarkably during these periods and close blood glucose control is important to establish. Education of patients with type I diabetes mellitus is key to preventing DKA and these patients should be taught to increase the frequency of their blood glucose monitoring and increase insulin appropriately in line with any increase in blood glucose. Failure to do this will result in glucose levels rising but the lack of insulin leads to increased production of glucagon, resulting in increased amounts of gluconeogenesis, glycogenolysis and lipolysis. A combination of the osmotic diuresis leading to dehydration and tissue hypoxia (leading to lactic acid production through anaerobic metabolism) and lipolysis leading to increased production of ketone bodies (which are inherently acidic) results in a florid metabolic acidosis, which may be severe enough to be life-threatening.

Treatment involves replacing any fluid losses with 0.9% normal saline (up to 6 L may be required in a 24-hour period) and commencement on a constant infusion of insulin at, for example, 6 units/hour in order to suppress ongoing ketogenesis (which will occur for some hours after blood glucose has been controlled).

Monitoring of the blood glucose and urinalysis for ketones is imperative to guide management and when the blood glucose drops to below 15 mmol/L then the infusion can be halved to 3 units/hour and 5% dextrose solution written up instead of saline as fluid replacement. Once the blood glucose is under adequate control, the urine is free from ketones and the patient is eating and drinking normally then consideration of normal insulin regimen is appropriate. If the patient is not yet fully established on eating and drinking then conversion to an insulin sliding scale (similar to but NOT the same as the insulin infusion as infusion rates are allowed to vary between 0.5 and 6 units) may be a step-down until oral intake is established. Potassium replacement should also be considered as although levels may appear normal acutely, when insulin infusion is started and resolution of acid–base deficits occur then potassium levels will inevitably fall and must be replaced accordingly.

8 a. Hypothyroidism may manifest with a plethora of features including constipation, bradycardia, hypothermia and confusion among other physical signs of thyroid dysfunction. Thyroid function tests should always be taken whilst investigating the cause of confusion in an elderly patient not otherwise known to be confused as extremes of both hyper- and hypofunction may lead to confusion. General reduction in mobility may be the root cause of falling in patients with hypothyroidism and should prompt investigation of thyroid dysfunction before more specialised falls investigation is performed. Electrocardiography may well reveal a sinus bradycardia, which along with an element of postural hypotension may well contribute to falling,

however, the cause of bradycardia should be investigated.

Echocardiography may be useful in detecting any clinically significant valvular disease, of which the most relevant to falls is aortic stenosis. The triad of symptoms typically associated with aortic stenosis (syncope, angina and dyspnoea) are often subtle in the elderly and often the only sign of severity is a fall leading to admission. CT scan of the head is part of the screen for confusion and reversible causes of dementia but may also reveal a subdural haematoma that may be contributing to or resulting from head injury sustained during a fall. In the presence of such florid clinical indices of thyroid dysfunction this should be considered only after blood tests have returned normal and the cause of confusion is still undiagnosed. Addison's disease (primary adrenocortical failure) may present in many different ways, however, the classical presentation is of hypotension, hyperkalaemia, hyponatraemia with nausea and vomiting. The short synacthen test is a specific test for Addison's disease and measurement of the cortisol level at baseline before and 30 minutes after injection of synthetic **ACTH** (hence the name!).

A rise of greater than 500 nmol/L at 30 minutes post-injection excludes Addison's disease. Treatment is of the underlying cause and replacement of steroids with prednisolone or hydrocortisone if oral intake is compromised.

9 e. Acute glaucoma, one of the most important ophthalmological emergencies, presents with a fixed dilated and often oval-shaped pupil.

129

Features of ophthalmological disease are as follows:

●

Acute glaucoma: Entire eye is red, both conjunctival and ciliary vessels are injected. Pupil is fixed, dilated and oval in shape, the intraocular pressure is high.

●

Iritis: Redness is most marked around the cornea and does not blanch on pressure. The pupil is small and fixed.

●

Conjunctivitis: Conjunctival vessels injected, blanch on pressure. Pupil is normal and reactive.

●

Subconjunctival haemorrhage: Bright red sclera with rim around limbus, pupil is normal.

10 b. Hypertension is a common cause of retinopathy and the history alone may aid in making a diagnosis that is further confirmed on fundoscopy. Classification schemes for hypertensive retinopathy wax and wane in popularity and may exist in the normal population as well as overlap with other syndromes such as diabetic retinopathy. The Scheie classification provides a simplified format from which to work from:

• *Grade 0*: Hypertensive but no visible retinal abnormalities

• *Grade I*: Arteriolar narrowing

• *Grade II*: Arteriolar narrowing with focal constriction

• *Grade III*: Diffuse narrowing with retinal haemorrhage

• *Grade IV*: Papilloedema and hard exudates

The changes seen in diabetic retinopathy (DR) are often

classified by the degree of retinopathy seen. However, this system is more useful clinically as local treatment, e.g. laser photocoagulation may be influenced by the degree of retinopathy.

The following classification represents a simplified format as schemes are in constant flux:

Background DR: Microaneurysms (dot) and microhaemorrhages (blot) and hard exudates.

Pre-proliferative DR: Cotton-wool spots and extensive blot haemorrhages.

• *Proliferative DR*: Neovascularisation.

Macular disease: Hard exudates encroaching on fovea or macular oedema.

Age-related macular degeneration (ARMD) can occur as 'dry' or 'wet' degeneration with the defining feature being the presence of choroidal neovascularisation (leading to 'wet' ARMD).

Although dry ARMD is by far the more commonly encountered type, wet ARMD is the more rapidly progressive and requires attention due to the accompanying visual deterioration that is seen. CMV retinitis usually occurs in the immunosuppressed and is sometimes seen in AIDS patients. It manifests as cotton-wool spots with flame haemorrhages often given the name 'pizza–pie' fundus because of its appearance. Ankylosing spondylitis usually presents with uveitis (inflammation of the components of the uveal tract; namely the iris, ciliary body and choroids) and is thought to occur in autoimmune disorders due to immune complex deposition in the uveal tract.

11 a. Approximately 45% of breast cancers occur in the upper outer quadrant of the breast. A quarter of cancers occur in the retro-areolar region with the lower inner quadrant being the least common site of tumours.

12 e. The majority of breast cancers are hormone sensitive. They are classified as oestrogen receptor positive or ER▣. For cancers that are hormone sensitive treatment may be commenced with

medications such as tamoxifen, which is an oestrogen receptor antagonist. With this in mind, risk factors for breast cancer can be thought of as those that increase the duration for which the body is producing hormones, e.g. those with an early menarche and late menopause. There is some controversy surrounding dairy produce in diet and whether there is any association with the development of breast cancer. There is at present no firm evidence to suggest that there is an association. Other risk factors for breast cancer include past history, use of oral contraceptives, never having breastfed and a family history.

13 b. Although all the investigations should be considered depending upon the chronicity of the swelling, the most important is to perform a joint aspiration. It is indefensible to miss a septic arthritis by not performing a diagnostic and simple tap in light of the above clinical signs. Septic arthritis will completely destroy a joint in a short space of time and the patient will head down the path of total joint replacement and potential lit-igation. Fluid should be sent for microscopy to look for organisms, cells and crystals (Note: gout and pseudogout), culture and sensitivities. Blood cultures are merited preferably prior to antibiotic therapy in light of the features of systemic infection, however, these should not be done in preference to aspiration.

Imaging of the knee joint is useful in due course to see the extent of damage if resolution is not achieved with antibiotic therapy.

14 d. Rheumatological disease exhibits a predilection for the female sex. Ankylosing spondylitis is one of the few conditions that goes against this trend being approximately 6 times more common in males than females in early teenage years and twice as common in males by 30 years of age. Typically the patient is a young male presenting with morning stiffness, reduced back movement with backpain and pain over the sacroiliac joints. Rheumatoid arthritis is unlikely for reasons of sex and age. Prolapsed intervertebral discs may present with symptoms of back and hip pain but would be again unlikely (but not infeasible) in a healthy 23-year-old man. Facet joint arthritis presents in middle-to-old age with pain especially on bending backwards as the facets rub against each other.

15 b. Rectal examination is avoided in neutropenic patients as trauma to the ano-rectum is easily manifested and may provide an easy access route to the bloodstream for gastrointestinal flora. Where possible these patients should be nursed in isolation in a side-room with full barrier nursing precautions.

These patients should be subjected to the minimal number of examinations and procedures and clinical staff should also be restricted to essential members only.

16 d. There is no association between iron deficiency anaemia and peripheral neuropathy. This finding is associated with a vitamin B12 deficiency. There are approximately 500 million cases of iron deficiency anaemia worldwide – it most commonly affects pre-menopausal women. The small bowel is responsible for absorption of iron, which is stored in the body in the form of ferritin. Signs of iron deficiency include koilonychias (spoon-shaped nails – both fingers and toes), angular stomatitis and glossitis. Other signs are associated with anaemias in general including fatigue and pallor.

17 d. Sickle cell disease is most commonly seen in patients of African, Arabian or Southern European descent. Carriers have one normal and one sickle gene and usually

132

remain asymptomatic. Those individuals homozygous for the sickle chain suffer with sickle cell disease. The red blood cells are of abnormal, sickle shape and therefore 'clog' smaller blood vessels resulting in ischaemia of distal tissues and associated pain. Clinical features include pallor as a result of the anaemia. Splenomegaly is seen in early disease but, as it progresses the spleen shrinks as due to the lack of blood supply. Bone crises are often predisposed by infection, cold or hypoxia, therefore the initial management of a sickle crisis is to apply oxygen and provide some symptomatic relief. Pigment gallstones are seen in the condition due to the haemolysis of the red blood cells. Leg ulcers are not a feature of this condition.

18 a. Endogenous depression, i.e. depression that occurs without an easily identifiable precipitant, was classically thought to be more resistant to treatment than exogenous (reactive) depression. This artificial classification, however, has lost favour among psychiatrists as the aetiology of depression becomes more multifactorial. Depression can be sub-classified according to severity and the components required to fulfil the diagnostic criteria for a major depressive episode are described below: At least five of the following, during the same 2-week period, representing a change from previous functioning; these must include either (1) or (2):

1. Depressed mood.

2. Diminished interest or pleasure (anhedonia).

3. Significant change in weight.

4. Insomnia or excessive sleepiness.

5. Psychomotor agitation or retardation.

6. Suicidal ideation or planned suicide.

7. Fatigue or loss of energy.

8. Feelings of worthlessness.

9. Reduced ability to concentrate.

The above symptoms must also not be associated with

signs of mania or excessive elevation of mood (leading more

towards a diagnosis of bipolar affective disorder), they must cause clinically significant distress of impairment of functioning and organic causes for symptomatology must be ruled out.

Symptoms must also not be associated with a grief response or bereavement. Females have been shown to be more prone to medication overdose and deliberate self-harm behaviour with males favouring more violent modes of suicide.

A lack of a confiding relationship has previously been described as a vulnerability factor for depression along with early maternal loss, greater than three children under 14 years at home and unemployment. These features are part of the Brown and Harris model of depression and have been postulated to be associated strongly with the development of depression.

Organic causes of depression or any change in mood or mental status must be ruled out prior to a diagnosis of psychiatric disease. This may include CT scan of the head and should include as routine blood glucose evaluation, thyroid hormones, vitamin B12 and folate levels, infection screen (including syphilis and, if indicated, HIV) and electrolyte and full blood count. Thyroid disease is the second most common endocrine disorder (after diabetes) and can present insidiously in the elderly population with features of depression or mood alteration.

19 c. Section 5(2) refers to a provision by the Mental Health Act for detention of an individual in the hospital against their own wishes for assessment of a mental health condition and is valid for 72 hours. It requires only one responsible medical officer and should only be used as a temporising measure until formal psychiatric evaluation can be carried out.

It would not be an appropriate course of action to allow this man to be discharged, either against medical advice (option D) or with follow-up with a community psychiatrist (option E), as he is likely to be a danger to himself or others and has already exhibited behaviour that would merit at least a brief period of assessment if not psychiatric treatment as an inpatient.

A Section 3 order refers to a detention order for a period of up to 6 months per Section 3 (i.e. it can be renewed) for treatment of a psychiatric condition. It is typically seen converted from a Section 2 where the assessment has been made and the decision to start treatment deemed appropriate. It requires two medical recommendations to be held valid.

Cuff and restraint under common law is not an appropriate modality to use in this case where a psychiatric diagnosis is suspected and would have to be justified on a case-by-case basis under the direct decision by a consultant physician.

134

20 c. In older males, a dilated abdominal aorta is relatively common finding. Other risk factors include with a family history of the complaint. In approximately 10% of cases an associated popliteal artery aneurysm will be found. Smaller aneurysms (below 4 cm) are considered to be benign and grow at a rate of 1–2 mm per year. The most feared complication of AAA's is rupture. Approximately 5% of aneurysms over 6 cm rupture spontaneously. Resection is usually advised in those aneurysms 5–6 cm in diameter. Complications of this surgery include renal failure since the renal artery ostia is often compressed during the procedure when the aorta is cross-clamped. Other complications include MI as coronary artery disease is usually present in those people with aortic compromise. As a result of cross clamping of the aorta the back pressure on the heart increases, which increases the workload of the heart. This, coupled with the metabolic stress that occurs when the legs are reperfused, may precipitate an MI.

21 d. Polycythaemia is commonly found in COPD patients and other respiratory diseases where gas transfer is reduced.

Chronic hypoxia stimulates the production of erythropoietin from the kidneys, which acts on the bone marrow to augment the oxygen carrying capacity of the blood. Usually this is the most important derangement that is found in the full blood count in the absence of an exacerbation.

22 a. This gentleman has a ventricular septar defect. This is an unusual but serious complication of MI, confirmed by echocardiography, and requires surgery to close the defect. On auscultation a pansystolic murmur is heard, which should raise suspicion, and the shortness of breath without radiological changes is caused by increased release of atrio-natriuretic peptide caused by increased pressure in the right atrium. Aortic regurgitation would give a diastolic murmur and heart failure would produce characteristic changes on the chest X-ray.

Dressler's syndrome is a late complication, occurring weeks to months after the initial insult and presents with recurrent pericarditis and pleural effusions associated with fever which doesn't fit this clinical presentation.

23 b. This boy has a classical history of a testicular torsion. This is usually torsion of the spermatic cord in a structurally abnormal testis. It is possible for it to occur in a structurally normal testis although, it is less common. This constitutes a surgical/urological emergency. Often there is a history of mild trauma or previous attacks of pain due to the torsion and spontaneous untwisting. The supply of the testis is from T10 sympathetic pathway which is why abdominal pain occurs. These patients require emergency surgery to correct and stabilise the torsion.

On occasions when the torsion has compromised the testicular blood supply for a long duration of time ischaemia may result which then requires an orchidectomy and treatment.

24 c. Testicular tumours are commonly found incidentally after minor trauma to the scrotum, the mass often mistakenly attributed to the trauma itself. Torsion of the testicular apparatus such as the hydatid of Morgagni is often heralded by pain and more rarely a blue spot on examination of the scrotum. In this particular case the diagnosis is made more suspicious by the scar in the groin, possibly attributed to previous surgery for undescended and maldescended testes, which are associated with testicular tumours. As a final point, seminoma is more commonly found in patients over 30 years of age than teratomas.

25 a. Dermatitis (eczema) is a common problem that often affects individuals whose line of work involves immersion in irritant substances such as bleach, shampoo, chemicals, washing up liquids and similar agents. Therefore one can predict with some accuracy a period of resolution from their dermatological problem when they are away from the workplace and hence irritant, such as during holiday periods. This type of dermatitis is sometimes referred to as extrinsic eczema to differentiate from intrinsic or atopic eczema. Lichen planus is typically associated with characteristic fine white lines that lie over the papules (Wickham's striae) and may affect the wrist. A chemical burn is a possibility, however, this does not usually present with an itchy rash. Porphyria cutanea tarda is a rare form of porphyria manifest as cutaneous photosensitivity. Psoriasis typically favours the extensor surfaces and usually presents as a non-itchy silver scale on an erythematous base.

26 c. Dermatitis herpetiformis forms crops of itchy blisters that are commonly found on elbows, knees and scalp. The itch can drive people to suicide and can be usually very effectively and with much gratitude relieved by oral dapsone. Dermatitis herpetiformis is associated with coeliac disease and as the risk of lymphoma is greatly increased by having both conditions, regular surveillance is recommended. Psoriasis does commonly affect the elbows but usually does not present with itch and eczema may present in such sites and with pruritus but is not strongly associated with coeliac disease. Scabies should always be kept in mind when considering itch, usually in children in the web spaces of the hands and feet. Track marks from the burrowing *Sarcoptes scabiei* mite can often be seen and harvested for microscopic diagnosis.

27 d. This girl is a legal minor in the eyes of the law and under common law is in the responsibility of her parents. However, a landmark legal case in 1985 (Gillick v West Norfolk and Wisbech Area Health Authority) brought to court by the parents of a teenage girl who was prescribed contraception without the know-ledge of her parents clarified the legal standpoint on medical treatment for those under the age of 16 years.

This standpoint is often referred to as Gillick competence (or the Fraser guidelines after the representative of the House of Lords who conceived the guidelines) in reference to this test case and reasons that young people in England and Wales (and Northern Island) under the age of 16 can consent to medical treatment if they have sufficient maturity and judgement to enable them fully to understand what is proposed. A similar law called the The Age of Legal Capacity (Scotland) Act 1991 exists in Scotland.

The Fraser guidelines are, however, open to interpretation by the agent assessing whether a minor is Gillick competent.

Thus it is the duty of the doctor or health care provider responsible for m172edical care and treatment of that minor to assess whether the ability to understand, retain and act upon information in an informed manner is present in those under the age of 16 years. If deemed the case then the minor assumes the same rights as any competent adult seeking medical treatment.

In this case referral to a family planning clinic is appropriate as it is both the girl's wish and will serve to provide support, education and contraceptive advice if sexual activity continues.

Counselling about sexual intercourse and contraceptive options is of vital importance in increasing the awareness of the merits and disadvantages of teenage pregnancy and the risk of sexually transmitted infection and blood-borne virus exposure.

Offering a sexually transmitted infection screen should occur in conjunction with counselling as she has been engaging in unprotected intercourse and most importantly she should also be encouraged to discuss the pregnancy and her feelings regarding sex with her parents. However, it must be stressed that any information shared with a health care professional can only be passed on to her parents with her express consent (if deemed Gillick competent).

28 a. In a young fit person the two most sensible treatment options include a surgical repair or a below knee cast with the foot in equinus position. After surgery, the re-rupture rate is 2–5% whilst it is 8–10% for those treated conservatively. The commonest site for rupture is 4–8 cm above the point of insertion. Characteristic signs of tendo Achilles rupture include difficulty in walking and standing on tip toes. There may also be a visible gap in the tendon and a positive Simmons test (no plantar flexion on squeezing the affected calf). If there is any doubt clinically, an ultrasound scan may be used to confirm the diagnosis. Conservative treatment is most appropriate for elderly people whilst younger and more active patients are usually managed with surgical repair. Infection is the biggest surgical complication involved with this procedure and since the Achilles tendon is quite superficial any wound infection may result in disrupting the integrity of the tendon repair.

29 a. The common peroneal nerve consists of branches of L4–S1. Its motor supply is to the anterior compartment of the calf including tibialis anterior and extensor hallucis longus. The sensory component supplies the 1st web space and the dorsum of the foot and front side of the leg. This nerve winds around the head of the tibia and in certain tibial plateau fractures its integrity may become compromised.

30 a. Sensitivity is defined as the number of disease and test positive (true positive) divided by the number of all the people with the disease. Represented as a formula this can be expressed as **a/(a ⬚ c)**. The table below can be used as reference for the following answers:

Test

Disease

Positive Negative

Positive a b

Negative c d

A test that has a high sensitivity is one that is appropriate to use as a screening test for a population as it will pull up few false negatives (high se**N**sitivity ⬚ few false **N**egatives) as most of the people who are disease positive will be 'caught' by the test as positive.

A test that has a high specificity, by comparison, should be used once enough individuals have been screened and will 'catch' those individuals who are disease and test negative (i.e. true negatives). This is good for weeding those people out who tested falsely positive in the screening test but are reassured to find out they are truly negative. It can be expressed as **d/(b ⬚ d)**.

Positive predictive value refers to the number of true positives who tested positive for the disease and can be expressed as **a/(a ⬚ b)**. As the accuracy of any test will increase with population size it follows that the positive predictive value of a test will increase the higher the prevalence of disease.

Negative predictive value refers to the number of true negatives who tested negative for the disease and can be expressed as **d/(c ⬜ d)**.

There were actually 140 false negatives in this case (box **c**) as these are defined as the number of people who are disease positive who test negative.

Finally this test should not be used as a screening test as the sensitivity is only 80.1% (**a/(a ⬜ c)**) which is not high enough to justify use as you would 'miss' approximately 20% of those with the disease as the test would not pick these people up.

31 b. The condition placenta praevia occurs when the placenta abnormally implants in the lower segment of the uterus.

Bleeding is usually painless unlike the other common cause of antepartum haemorrhage, abruptio placentae (placental abruption). Physical signs are usually few. Breech or oblique presentation is occasionally seen due to the mechanical obstruction to birth canal outflow. Routine ultrasound scans may over-estimate the prevalence of this condition as the lower segment grows cephalically late in the last trimester and it is estimated that up to 10% of placentae are low-lying before 37 weeks. Cervical cancer would otherwise be a diagnosis not to be dismissed, however, as cervical smears are usually recommended as part of antenatal care, this makes this option unlikely. Placenta accreta is usually encountered at Caesarean section, often with catastrophic effect, and does not usually present with antepartum haemorrhage.

32 c. This lady has suffered a deep vein thrombosis. Risk factors for deep vein thrombosis include:

- Past history

- Pregnancy

- Malignancy

- Antiphospholipid syndrome

- Oral contraceptive pill use

- Nephrotic syndrome

- Recent surgery

- Pelvic mass

• Recent childbirth

• Obesity

Whilst she has no past history she is pregnant and therefore has a pelvic mass! In pregnancy, patients may be reluctant to take anticoagulants. The diagnosis should be confirmed as soon as possible and if for any reason there is a delay, treatment dose of a low molecular weight heparin should be administered.

33 c. Cystic fibrosis is characterised by a defect in a chloride channel transporter and is usually due to single amino acid substitution at position 508. Children usually suffer from multiple recurrent chest infections (usually due to *Pseudomonas*) failure to thrive and malabsorption. Cystic fibrosis should be at the forefront of a differential diagnosis of any chest problems and failure to thrive in any infant. PAS positive macrophages refers to a finding in Whipple's disease caused by the Gram positive rod *Tropheryma whippelii*. Whipple's disease usually causes malabsorption in men over 50 years old. Cobblestone appearance is a typical finding on barium enema in Crohn's disease – a disease affecting any part of the gastrointestinal system, unlike ulcerative colitis. A double bubble on abdominal X-ray is occasionally seen associated with Down's syndrome due to duodenal atresia. Abnormal bone marrow cytology refers to the possibility of a haematological malignancy such as acute myelogenous leukaemia and unlikely to present in this manner.

34 b. The growth of male breast tissue, known as gynaecomastia, is a normal finding in the neonate due to maternal oestrogens and in the pubertal boy and elderly male due to the changing ratio of testosterone to oestrogens in these age groups. This is not a typical finding that would be consistent with non-accidental injury and therefore a referral to social services would be inappropriate. Referral to a breast surgeon and needle aspiration are also unjustified in this case and may even be deleterious to growing breast tissue. Short course prednisolone is also unwarranted and is not indicated in cases of gynaecomastia.

35 d. The transverse colon is spared many of the complications that are commonly seen in the sigmoid colon; the site of most pathology in the gastrointestinal tract. A host of conditions including diverticulitis, volvulus, colorectal carcinoma and angiodysplasia to mention but a few afflict this area. Ruptured aortic aneurysms are most often seen in older men, however, the clinical picture of upper abdominal pain, raised inflammatory markers and a high amylase in a clinically unstable patient should prompt investigation to rule out this fatal condition. Pancreatitis is one of the most likely causes of the above clinical picture and an amylase less than the often quoted limit of 4 times normal (360 IU/L) does not exclude this common condition.

36 c. Rigler's sign is a radiographic finding of bowel perforation.

It manifests as a dual-enhanced image of the bowel due to the presence of air in the peritoneum and in the lumen of the bowel. Murphy's sign is positive when pain is elicited over the right upper quadrant when two fingers are placed here and the patient asked to breathe in. An inflamed gallbladder will cause the patient to catch his or her breath. Rovsing's sign relates to pain felt in the right iliac fossa when pressure is applied to the left iliac fossa and is associated with appendicitis.

Kerr's sign is pain felt in the shoulder tips associated most classically with ruptured ectopic pregnancy. This pain is referred pain from blood irritating the diaphragm and emphasises the common embryological relationship between the motor innervation of the diaphragm (C3, C4 and C5) and the sensory dermatome supplying the shoulder tips (C4). Trousseau's sign in the context of abdominal disease relates to crops of tender nodules affecting blood vessels (*thrombophlebitis migrans*) often associated with pancreatic malignancy.

37 d. Bile leak is a recognised complication of hepatobiliary surgery and presents within days post-operatively. Bile is a potent irritant to the peritoneum causing a chemical biliary peritonitis associated with rising biliary enzymes and bilirubin. Conservative management will often suffice for minor leaks, however, surgical intervention is the definitive treatment in severe cases.

Accidental ligation of the common bile duct is a rare but catastrophic complication of cholecystectomy, however, this is not routinely seen in cyst fenestration. Cholecystitis presents with a similar clinical picture but does not usually present with such marked derangement of liver enzymes without the co-existent bile duct involvement seen in biliary colic. Propofol is commonly used as an anaesthetic induction agent and although associated with hepatotoxicity in large doses would not normally cause significant hepatic injury. Biliary sepsis is always a high risk with hepatobiliary surgery but presents characteristically with relatively normal liver enzymes and signs of clinical sepsis.

38 a. Pulmonary embolus is an often overlooked risk of laparoscopic procedures. During surgery the peritoneum is insufflated with carbon dioxide to a pressure of around 15 mmHg. Occlusion of the venous system draining through the abdomen including the great vessels has been reported to increase the incidence of post-operative venous thromboembolism. Thromboembolic deterrent stockings (TEDS) are recommended for 4 weeks with daily injection of subcutaneous low-molecular weight heparin for any patient who has recently undergone laparoscopic procedures. Pulmonary embolus is associated with pleuritic chest pain, tachycardia, the often quoted, rarely seen deep S wave in lead I, deep Q wave in lead III and inverted T wave in lead III (S1,Q3,T3), with haemoptysis or silently. Beware the elderly on beta-blocking medication who do not mount a tachycardia; a useful warning sign of pulmonary embolus!

39 b. Fibrin degradation products (D-dimer) is a test useful only in the process of ruling out a pulmonary embolus. A negative result predicts a high likelihood of absence of pulmonary embolus; a positive result is almost meaningless diagnostically.

D-dimers are expected to rise post-operatively and thus should not form the first line of investigation for a suspected pulmonary embolus. Arterial blood gases and electrocardiography are invaluable for the investigation of dyspnoea for both quantifying the respiratory compromise and in stratifying the differential to either cardiac or respiratory causes. Chest radiographs may demonstrate pneumonic processes or pneumothoraces and form part of the standard investigation of breathlessness.

CT-PA forms the most definitive imaging in cases of suspected pulmonary embolus but may return equivocal results in the presence of pre-existing lung pathology.

40 c. Inguinal hernias present the greatest diagnostic challenge when defining the subtype of hernia; indirect hernias were often said to be controlled by pressure over the internal (deep) inguinal ring at a point 1–2 cm above the femoral pulse once reduced. However, this clinical distinction is frequently inaccurate in even the most experienced hands. A more useful definition is that direct hernias pass medially to the inferior epigastric artery with indirect hernias passing laterally. This can be neatly summed up as 'MDs don't Lie' (**M**edial **D**irect, **L**ateral **I**ndirect). Confusion between inguinal and femoral hernias can be avoided by remembering that inguinal hernias present above and medial to the pubic tubercle with femoral hernias presenting below and lateral. Spighelian hernias are located at the lateral border of the posterior rectus sheath, passing through the arcuate line to present as a mass in the lower abdominal wall. Ventral hernias are often seen in the elderly and are associated with a widening of the recti muscles (divari-cation of the recti).

41 b. Acute exacerbations of asthma can be defined as severe or life-threatening. Criteria for diagnosis are as follows:

Severe attack

142

- unable to complete sentences

- respiratory rate of greater than 25/minute

- heart rate greater than 110 beats per minute

- PEFR of less than 50% of predicted

Life-threatening

- cyanosis, very poor respiratory effort

- silent chest

- bradycardia and hypotension

- PEFR

↕33% predicted

Arterial blood sampling will show normal or high PCO2 and

PO2 less than 8kPa.

In any case of asthma exacerbation a chest X-ray should be ordered to exclude a pneumothorax and to look for a concurrent pneumonia. The principles for management of exacerbations can be remembered by the mnemonic 'O SHIT';

O: Oxygen

S: Salbutamol

H: Hydrocortisone (or prednisolone)

I: Inhaled steroids

T: Theophylline (be aware of risks of toxicity – if not already on regular theophyllines will need a loading dose)

Magnesium is now used in acute asthma and the use of theophyllines is reducing. Check with your trust about local policy.

42 e. Whilst this lady has a strong history of asthma it is important to exclude other causes of shortness of breath. Anaphylaxis refers to a severe allergic reaction including both dermal and systemic signs and symptoms. The full-blown syndrome includes urticaria with occasional angioedema with hypotension and bronchospasm. Anaphylaxis is mediated by IgE and symptoms and signs are caused by rapid onset of increased secretion from mucous membranes, increased bronchial smooth muscle tone, reduced vascular smooth muscle tone and increased capillary permeability occur after exposure to an offending substance.

Pneumothorax is a collection of gas in the pleural space resulting in collapse of the lung on the affected side. A tension pneumothorax can be a life-threatening condition caused by air within the pleural space that is under pressure. This causes displacement of mediastinal structures which in turn compromises car-diopulmonary function.

Tracheal obstruction or a massive pulmonary embolus will understandably cause acute onset shortness of breath. Stridor may be a clue in airway obstruction and a history of risk factors should be sought in a suspected pulmonary embolus. An upper respiratory tract infection should not present acutely.

43 e. Pulmonary embolus and deep vein thrombosis risk should be assessed in all patients who present with pleuritic pain and shortness of breath. Patients post-surgery, especially hip surgery, obese patients, malignant disease, immobility and the oral contraceptive pill all increase the likelihood of a venous thromboembolism. Carotid massage would be completely contraindicated in this woman as she is hypotensive. It is useful as a first-line manoeuvre in cases of supraventricular tachycardia once the absence of a carotid bruit has been established.

Frusemide is useful in cases of heart failure in the presence of relatively normal renal function. CT with pulmonary angiography is the gold standard for diagnosing but not treating pulmonary embolus but is not even an option in this case due to this woman's unstable condition.

44 b. Intramuscular adrenaline injection of 1 mL of 1:1000 adrenaline is the recommended treatment for suspected anaphylaxis.

Note that this dose differs from the 1:10000 intravenous (i.v.) injection dose of adrenaline used in cardiac arrest. The clues to a severe allergic reaction are manifold from the history; severe shortness of breath occurs secondary to oedema of the upper airway and larynx and his medications reveal an atopic predisposition. Laryngeal mask airway and endotracheal intubation would be possibilities if adrenaline did not work as a first line or if airway control was an issue. Nebulised salbutamol and i.v.

hydrocortisone would provide some relief for airway oedema but are not as effective as adrenaline in the acute management of anaphylaxis.

45 b. This question is slightly controversial as there are two possible answers that might be considered depending on the clinical situation. This patient has two main problems; as he is drowsy he is not likely to protect his airway and thus is at risk of aspiration, and on clinical examination he has evidence of a right-sided tension pneumothorax. Most clinicians would consider attempting a procedure such as needle thoracocentesis to drain a tension pneumothorax before securing an airway. A nasopharyngeal airway is contraindicated due to the complex facial fractures as the risk of basal skull fracture is high. An emergency tracheostomy is a last resort attempt to secure an airway and can be avoided by early intubation if airway management is likely to become difficult. Chest drain insertion is not the recommended procedure for releasing a tension pneumothorax.

46 b. Advanced Parkinson's disease can result in many features including a mask-like facial appearance and a difficulty in swallowing. This patient suffered an aspiration pneumonia. The commonest site for an aspiration pneumonia, or indeed inhalation of a foreign body, is the right lower lobe of the lung. This is due to the anatomy of the right main bronchus being more vertical than the left due to the positioning of the heart. Parkinson's disease is not known to be closely associated with heart failure.

Atypical pneumonias are usually widespread and provide more generalised signs than those described above.

47 c. INR (International Normalised Ratio) is derived from the prothrombin time, which is then normalised against a laboratory standard to give values that are interpretable and stand-ardised wherever the tests are taken. The INR is a very specific and sensitive indicator of liver damage and is the investigation of choice when assessing liver function (although many laboratories persist with using the incorrect liver function test terminology when assaying levels of liver transaminases). Albumin is also a product of liver synthesis and can be expected to fall with chronic liver diseases. Glycaemic control is also regulated in a large part by the liver and hypoglycaemia due to impaired gluconeogenesis and glycogen storage is often a complication of patients with advanced liver impairment. AST and ALT are useful markers of acute liver insult such as hepatitis, however, they are not well correlated with the degree of liver failure. Alkaline phosphatase and bilirubin are often associated with obstruction of the biliary system and will often rise in obstructive jaundice preferentially to the transaminases. Fibrinogen is a useful indicator of consumption and turnover of clotting products and can be low in disseminated intravascular coagulation (DIC) and venous thromboembolism (VTE).

48 b. This woman has developed *Clostridium difficile* diarrhoea, which is associated with pseudomembranous colitis. It is particularly a complication of clindamycin use but few antibiotics are completely free of this side-effect. Treatment is with either metronidazole or vancomycin for more seriously ill patients. Her blood results can be explained by dehydration due to fluid and electrolyte loss from the gastrointestinal tract. Intravenous potassium replacement is rarely indicated in patients with hypokalaemia and in fact in inexperienced hands may be extremely dangerous due to cardiac arrhythmias. Diuresis is not indicated as this woman is in negative fluid balance and the addition of amoxicillin is unlikely to be effective at treating *C. difficile* diarrhoea. Blood is not needed in this case for fluid replacement; 0.9% normal saline is adequate.

49 d. Autoimmune hepatitis (AIH) tends to affect young- to middle-aged women and may present acutely with features of hepatitis or more insidiously with features of chronic liver disease. Extra-hepatic involvement is common with rash, arthralgia and arthritis accompanying more constitutional features of hepatitis such as nausea, malaise, vomiting and loss of appetite as well as weight loss. An interesting finding is that many women experience amenorrhoea and the clinical picture of a young woman of childbearing age with vomiting, loss of appetit and some abdominal pain can easily lead to misdiagnosis if an accurate history is not taken. Antibody screens are useful in making the diagnosis and a dichotomy is classically described between those individuals with Type I and Type II AIH:

• *Type I*: Involvement of antinuclear antibodies (ANA) with or without antismooth muscle antibodies (SMA).

• *Type II*: Mainly children involved and with liver/kidney microsomal Type I antibodies (LKM1).

Budd–Chiari syndrome presents with acute epigastric pain and shock and is due to occlusion of the hepatic vein. It presents rapidly and would not fit the clinical picture in this case. Viral hepatitis is an option to be considered in any young person with a tender right upper quadrant especially in the face of mild jaundice and hepatomegaly and risk assessment should be carried out for blood-borne viruses and possibly hepatitis serology.

McArdle's syndrome is a glycogen storage disease (Type V) and presents with muscular pain after exercise due to deficiency in myophosphorylase. A muscle biopsy is diagnostic. A useful mnemonic for remembering the rare disorders of glycogen storage is 'Very Poor Carbohydrate Metabolism' standing for Von Gierke's disease, Pompé's disease, Cori's disease and McArdle's disease.

50 a. Pharyngeal pouches occur more commonly in men than women and in the elderly. The features described above are classically associated with the presence of a pharyngeal pouch.

There have been instances of rupture of the pouch, most usually at oesophogastroduodenoscopy (OGD) if there has not been a significant suspicion of pouch disease, however, most cases are diagnosed early and surgically amenable to excision and repair. The pouch forms at an anatomical weakness between the inferior pharyngeal muscle complex posteriorly,

known as Killian's dehiscence. Diagnostically is it best seen on contrast swallow where the pouch is clearly delineated.

Plummer–Vinson syndrome describes iron-deficiency anaemia and dysphagia caused by the formation of a keratinised web.

Features associated with iron deficiency such as koilonychia (spoon-shaped nails) and atrophic glossitis may be rarely seen.

The post-cricoid web is a direct but very rare consequence of severe iron-deficiency anaemia. Chagas' disease was described by a Brazilian physician who described the characteristic

symptoms of achalsia (failure of the oesophageal cardia to relax) in the South American population with *Trypanosoma cruzi* infection. Contrast swallow shows the level of obstruction often with hugely dilated and poorly functioning proximal oesophagus.

A failure of neuromuscular co-ordination is thought to be the pathogenesis behind the disease. Mallory–Weiss tear often follows a large meal and binge-drinking leading to a small linear tear in the oesophageal mucosa. Oesophageal carcinoma presents with progressive dysphagia for solids then liquids often with florid constitutional signs of cancer.

51 b. ERCP would be the next most appropriate investigation as this man has the symptoms and blood test picture most likely to be primary sclerosing cholangitis (PSC). The association between ulcerative colitis and PSC is well recognised and up to 75% of patients with PSC may have inflammatory bowel disease. Liver biopsy is a useful investigation to confirm the diagnosis in cases with equivocal or borderline investigative results and shows a characteristic 'onion-skin' appearance to the intrahepatic biliary system. ERCP in most cases will make the diagnosis with a 'beaded' appearance due to alternating section of dilatation and stricture of the bile ducts. CT scan may detect areas of liver damage due to chronic backpressure from strictured bile ducts but is far less superior at imaging the biliary tree than magnetic resonance cholangiopancreatography (MRCP). Colonoscopy is useful for detecting inflammatory bowel conditions in patients who present with abdominal pain and change of bowel habit but may have additional benefit in screening for colorectal cancer, which is increased in risk by PSC. Plain abdominal radiography is only of benefit in the diagnosis of complications of inflammatory bowel conditions such as bile duct fistula (aerobilia) and bowel obstruction due to stricture as the most important.

52 c. The clinical picture is one of carcinoid syndrome secondary to a carcinoid tumour. The syndrome of facial flushing,

watery diarrhoea, abdominal pain and cardiac abnormalities imply hepatic metastases of a carcinoid tumour. Common sites in the bowel are terminal ileum, rectum and appendix (25% of all tumours), however, involvement of other organs such as ovaries or testes have been reported. Diagnosis is elegantly made from the clinical picture and 24-hour collection of urine for levels of 5-HIAA, a metabolite of 5-HT

(serotonin) that is postulated to be responsible for the cardiac manifestations of the disease and profuse watery diarrhoea. 24-hour urine collection for protein is useful in cases of renal disease where the amount of proteinuria can be quantified. Urine and plasma osmolalities are usually taken together in the diagnosis of disorders of free water clearance such as the syndrome of inappropriate ADH (SIADH). A low plasma sodium is seen in the face of inappropriately high urine osmolality indicating free water retention. Fluid restriction may be used to bring the level of sodium up slowly. Too rapid correction of plasma sodium is associated with the development of central pontine myelinolysis – a catastrophic shrinking in the size of brain cells due to rapid osmolarity shifts, which may be fatal. 24-hour urine collection for the presence of VMA (metabolites of catecholamines) may be helpful in making the diagnosis of phaeochromocytoma, a rare catecholamine producing tumour. 90% of tumours are in the adrenal medulla, 90% benign and 90% of these unilateral.

53 b. This gentleman provides a good history that raises suspicion of subarachnoid haemorrhage (SAH). He requires an urgent CT scan of his brain to rule this out and to assess for raised intracranial pressure. This is usually indicated in order to proceed with a lumbar puncture to assess for xanthochromia as up to 10% of SAH can be missed on CT scan alone. An MRI scan of this gentleman's brain would provide a detailed view of his cerebral parenchyma, although this is not the first-line investigation in this case. The history given includes no mention of fever, therefore looking for a systemic infective cause with blood cultures is unnecessary. Neurological observations and regular analgesia, although important, are unlikely to aid with the diagnosis and therefore are not first-line considerations.

54 c. Lesions of the cerebellum provide characteristic signs that can be remembered by the mnemonic 'DANISH P':

D: dysdiadochokinesis

A: ataxia

N: nystagmus

I: intention tremor

S: slurred speech

H: hypotonia

P: past pointing

This lady's lesion is in the cerebellar vermis as she has bilateral signs of cerebellar disease. Lesions of the bilateral basal ganglia would be incredibly unusual and provide Parkinson's-like features including a rest tremor. A lesion of the left temporo-parietal lobe would provide a dysphasia (assuming this is her dominant hemisphere) and some visual field defects in addition to hemisensory neglect. Lesions of the frontal lobe would result in personality changes and dysphasia – not in keeping with the clinical details in this case.

55 c. Of the listed investigations, CT scan is the most important to obtain. This lady is displaying signs of a vascular event; distinguishing between an infarct or haemorrhage is vital and this can be done by CT scan. Although an INR level will give us vital information about her anticoagulation state, in the short term this is not imperative. A carotid duplex scan could be a helpful adjunct to a cardiovascular examination in identifying a cause of an ischaemic episode if that transpires to be the case.

Electrocardiogram and echocardiogram would again identify a cardiac cause of any emboli if the CT scan showed an infarct, however, these are not first-line investigations.

56 b. This patient has Wilson's disease. It is an autosomal recessive disorder affecting the lenticular nuclei (globus pallidus and puta-men) and the liver, hence the description of hepatolenticular degeneration. Copper deposits can also be seen in the cornea scleral junction. Copper and caeruloplasmin screening should reveal the diagnosis which can be confirmed with the positive family history. Wilson's disease should be considered in patients with acute mental state changes or impaired mental development for their age. Porphyria is most likely to present with colicky abdominal pain, vomiting and fever. It is a low penetrant autosomal dominant condition. Glycogen storage disorders e.g. Hunter's syndrome, usually present as gargoylism in children.

Presentation of Parkinsonism at this age, unless drug-related, is rare and the symptoms and signs are not identified in this case.

57 a. Superficial temporal arteritis is 'never' seen in patients this age.

It is a disease of the over 55s and is more prevalent in women than men. There is a 25% association with polymyalgia rheumatica and symptoms of scalp and temporal artery tenderness, e.g. on brushing hair, pain whilst eating and most drastically sudden blindness in one eye. Thus any suspicion of superficial temporal arteritis should prompt immediate twice daily 40–60mg prednisolone until the diagnosis has been disproven.

All the other causes of headache are commonly experienced in the general practice setting and could reliably be attributable for the pattern of symptoms exhibited by this patient.

58 d. Papilloedema is congestion of the optic disc invariably associated with raised intracranial pressure. It is most often bilateral.

General features reflect the underlying disease process but a choked disc is characteristic, though differentiation from papillitis may be difficult.

In the acute setting vision is rarely affected but peripheral vision may be lost in chronic cases where it is frequently accompanied by transient visual obscurations. Papilloedema results from raised intracranial pressure in which the subarachnoid space surrounding the optic nerve is patent e.g. papil-loedema is not necessarily a consequence of raised intracranial pressure.

Causes include:

• Intracranial space-occupying lesions – tumours, especially of the posterior fossa due to restricted space; cerebral abscesses; subdural haematoma.

• Any condition that results in hydrocephalus in an adult, e.g. subarachnoid haemorrhage, meningitis, head injury.

• Venous sinus thrombosis due to congestion.

• Benign intracranial hypertension – most likely in patients with visual complaints but otherwise normal.

• Malignant hypertension – bilateral with other signs of hypertensive neuropathy.

• Central retinal venous occlusion, ischaemic optic neuropathy, optic neuritis – unilateral with sudden loss of vision.

• Chronic carbon dioxide retention.

Other rare causes include:

• Metabolic:

– Hypoparathyroidism

– Diabetic ketoacidosis

– Chronic carbon dioxide retention

– Obesity.

• Haematological – anaemia, leukaemia.

• Toxic – tetracycline, lead, oral progestational agents, corticosteroid withdrawal.

• Spinal cord tumours.

59 e. The condition described is typical of retroperitoneal fibrosis (peri-aortitis). It is an autoimmune condition where there is progressive fibrosis surrounding the aorta, into which the ureters become embedded causing renal obstruction, failure and retention. Methysergide has a particular association and may still be seen in use for resistant migraine. Paracetamol can lead to acute tubular necrosis as an adverse side effect and acyclovir may cause crystal deposition in cases of dehydration. Gold injections should also be monitored regularly for renal side-effects by follow-up urinalysis for proteinuria. Rosiglitazone must be used with caution in patients with pre-existing renal impairment but itself has few renal side-effects in normal kidneys.

60 d. Tuberculosis should always be in the forefront of the differential diagnosis of a patient who has recently come from a developing country, who exhibits weight loss and fever. This presentation is not classic for tuberculosis, however, the presence of a constitutional upset with a sterile pyuria is good enough cause to investigate for the disease. Treating for a urinary tract infection with antibiotics or antifungals is not correct without first excluding growth of alcohol and acid fast bacilli (AAFB) in culture specimens. An intravenous urogram may be necessary down the line to investigate any specific blockage to the urinary tract but a chest X-ray is mandatory for any suspicion of tuberculosis so prompt treatment and barrier nursing precautions can take place if necessary. Cystoscopy is unlikely to be helpful as there has been no mention of any haematuria and may be considered at a later stage if indirect imaging is inconclusive.

Extended matching questions

61 b. This lady is suffering from a pneumonia; this can be associated with chest pain. Risk factors for her developing chest infections include the fact that she has a history of lung disease and that she resides in a nursing home. Sedentary lifestyles are more often associated with acquiring infections particularly in institutionalised patients.

62 e. Bornholm's disease is a post viral illness that is associated with costochondritis. Patients describe a chest pain that can be recreated by sternal pressure, similar to Tietze's syndrome or idiopathic costochondritis, but on further questioning its incidence closely follows a viral illness.

63 g. The clue in this scenario is the recent addition of diclofenac into his medication list. The history obtained from this gentleman suggests a diagnosis of GORD or gastro-oesophageal reflux disease. Exacerbation of his symptoms on lying flat suggest a gastric association and deficiency in the distal oesophageal sphincter. The nausea associated with this pain could be associated with cardiac pain but in the context of this history we can be reassured that the likely cause of this gentleman's pain is GI in origin.

64 h. Acute onset chest pain which is described as radiating to the back is characteristic of aortic dissection. Aortic dissection is defined as separation of the layers within the aortic wall.

Tears in the intimal layer result in the propagation of dissection (proximally or distally) secondary to blood entering the intima-media space. Aortic dissection is more common in males than in females, with a male-to-female ratio of 2:1. The condition commonly occurs in persons in the sixth and seventh decades of life. Patients with Marfan's syndrome present earlier, usually in the third and fourth decades of life.

DeBakey classified aortic dissection into three types, as follows:

- *Type I*: The intimal tear occurs in the ascending aorta, but the descending aorta

152

is also involved.

- *Type II*: Only the ascending aorta is involved.

- *Type III*: Only the descending aorta is involved:

—

Type IIIA involves the descending aorta that originates distal to the left subclavian artery and extends as far as the diaphragm.

—

Type IIIB involves the descending aorta below the diaphragm.

The pain of aortic dissection may be distinguished from the pain of acute myocardial infarction by its abrupt onset, although the presentations of the two conditions overlap to some degree. Aortic dissection should be strongly considered in patients with symptoms and signs suggestive of myocardial infarction but without classic ECG findings.

65 c. Risk factors for pulmonary embolus include immobility, malignancy, post-operative period for abdominal or pelvic surgery, lower limb fractures, previous thrombo-embolic disease, pregnancy and hip or knee replacements. In addition to these there are further minor risk factors including long distance travel, use of combined oral contraceptive pill or hormone replacement therapy. In the case in question, this lady is 1 week in the post-operative period for having a knee replacement. The mention in the case of right calf swelling, progressing to chest pain exacerbated by inspiration is a classical description of a pulmonary embolus.

A ventilation/perfusion scan or a CT pulmonary angiogram should be organised to confirm the diagnosis and treatment dose anticoagulation should be commenced as soon as the diagnosis is suspected and if confirmed this should be replaced with warfarin.

66 a. Cushing's syndrome manifests clinically with a plethora of clinical signs due to excess amounts of corticosteroid. The typical clinical picture is of an obese patient who exhibits a moon face appearance, abnormal fatty pads over the neck and upper back leading to the classical buffalo hump with easily bruised and paper thin skin. Hypertension and diabetes mellitus are commonly found due to both the mineralocorticoid and glucocorticoid effects of excess corticosteroid and a picture of hypernatraemia and hypokalaemia provides a clue to the pathology in the face of a strong clinical suspicion. Cushing's syndrome can be as a result of Cushing's disease, which describes the above clinical findings as a consequence of a primary pituitary neoplasm (usually adenoma). Other ACTH-dependent causes may be due to an ectopic focus of ACTH secretion such as a small-cell carcinoma of the lung. ACTH-independent causes include a primary adrenocortical tumour such as an adenoma or commonly exogenous steroid use such as that seen often in those requiring steroid immunosuppression for transplants or autoimmune disease.

67 g. Hypothyroidism may present in the elderly with very non-specific signs and should be considered in the differential of anyone presenting with confusion (so-called part of the 'dementia' screen) and general deterioration with no readily identifiable cause. One of the most common endocrine disturbances alongside diabetes mellitus, it should not be missed as a cause of a range of symptoms from neurological signs, typically bradykinesia, reduced deep tendon reflexes and parasthesias from nerve entrapment (especially carpal tunnel syndrome) to abdominal pain from chronic constipation to mental disturbance manifest as confusion and apparent memory impairment. Other subtle signs of hypothyroidism include loss of the outer one-third of the eyebrows with male-pattern frontal balding, hypothermia (leading to the aptly named 'granny's tartan' – erythema *ab igne* from sitting close to or being in close contact with a source of heat such as a fire, electric heater or hot-water bottle), bradycardia and dry, coarse skin. Thyroid function tests are usually diagnostic and demonstrate a low free T4 with a compensatory high TSH in primary hypothyroidism. Very occasionally a low TSH and a low free T4 may be seen in the context of panhypopituitarism and assay of levels of sex hormones, ACTH and other pituitary hormones will confirm the diagnosis.

68 c. Diabetes mellitus can often present in a similar fashion to other endocrine diseases and thus it is important that investigations be interpreted in the correct fashion. Loss of weight, fatigue, polydipsia and polyuria are features of not only diabetes mellitus but also diabetes insipidus (DI) (resulting from to loss of free water due to an inability to secrete or respond to vasopressin and thus be able to concentrate urine). Occasionallyhysterical polydipsia manifests with the above clinical features and can be difficult to clinically distinguish from DI. In this case performing urine electrolyte and osmolality studies can differentiate between these two very different conditions; in DI there is secretion of free water and thus urine osmolality is very low, however, in hysterical polydipsia urine osmolality is normal as intake is matched by output keeping an overall iso-tonic balance to osmolality. Clues in the scenario suggesting a diagnosis of diabetes mellitus are the concurrent infection (that raises stress hormone levels e.g. cortisol causing an increase in blood glucose levels), the high urine osmolality (due to high glucose load as the renal tubular threshold for glucose absorption has been exceeded) and the very high plasma osmolality.

154

This can be approximated thus:

Posm ~ 2(Na⁫) ⁫ K⁫ ⁫ urea ⁫ glucose → units ⁫ mOsm/L

Plugging in the values for sodium, potassium and urea leaves the remaining component (glucose) at 20.1. This high glucose in the absence of any previous history of diabetes mellitus suggests a type II manifestation of high blood sugar; hyperosmolar hyperglycaemic state (previously hyperosmolar non-ketotic coma, HONK). Urine dipstick will confirm the presence of heavy ketonuria (suggestive of diabetic ketoacidosis (DKA) or an element of HONK/DKA overlap) and an arterial blood gas would demonstrate the pH. As a general rule, any event such as surgery, illness or even myocardial infarction can manifest clinically in addition to the primary event with features of high blood glucose control, which may then progress to hyperosmolar hyperglycaemic state or DKA.

69 b. The diagnosis of acromegaly can often be very subtle with those closest to the patient often bringing the changes to attention. It is often helpful to look at old photographs if there is a suspicion of acromegaly as coarsening of features, protrusion of the jaw (prognathism) and change in clothing or shoe size may all point to a retrospective diagnosis. Most often due to a pituitary adenoma (80% macroadenoma, 20% microadenoma) visual symptoms may be a complaint alongside headache and even bedside visual field testing may reveal a defect, commonly a bitemporal hemianopia (tunnel vision). Sausage fingers (leading to an inability to wear rings), greasy coarse skin and a thickening of the forehead are all signs of growth-hormone excess that characterises acromegaly. Trans-sphenoidal hypo-physectomy is usually employed as a treatment modality, sometimes in conjunction with medical therapy to reduce the size of a very large macroadenoma or surgically incompletely resected tumour.

70 e. Phaeochromocytoma is a rare tumour of the sympathetic nervous system notable for the production of catecholamines. Tumours may be adrenal or extra-adrenal and occur in both children and adults. The 'Rule of 10' mnemonic is a helpful way of remembering that phaeochromocytomas are **10%** ectopic, **10%** malignant and **10%** multiple. Symptoms may often be mistaken for anxiety attacks or cardiac in origin as palpitations, tremors, severe anxiety with no basis and chest pain may all be manifestations of the tumour. Severe hypertension is commonly associated and this may prompt more serious investigation of otherwise subtle symptomatology. Plasma metanephrines (metabolic products of catecholamine pathways) is the most sensitive investigation but a useful screening tool is the 24-hour urine collection for metanephrines and catecholamines. Imaging modalities should be used only on the basis of a strong clinical suspicion and/or biochemical evidence of a catecholamine disturbance as the incidence of adrenal mass (so-called incidentaloma) found on imaging has been estimated to be around the order of 7% in the elderly population.

MRI scanning of the abdomen is the preferred and most sensitive and specific modality and thus should be employed after positive biochemical tests have been confirmed.

71 b. Rheumatoid arthritis affects females 3 times more commonly than males. Its peak age of onset is between the ages of 30 and 50 years old. It can be described as a symmetrical polyarthropathy affecting both small and large joints. Common symptoms are swollen, painful, stiff hands and feet, worse in the mornings. Patients may also describe a recent history of constitutional symptoms and fatigue. Patients with suspected rheumatoid arthritis should always be referred to a rheuma-tologist for commencement of disease modifying drugs as soon as the diagnosis is confirmed in order to reduce the amount of joint damage sustained.

72 a. In acute gout there is often severe pain, redness and swelling in the affected joint. The metatarsophalangeal joint of the big toe is most commonly affected. Deposition of sodium monou-rate crystals in the joint space are responsible for the symptoms and attacks may be precipitated by trauma, surgery, starvation or commencement of diuretics. Risk factors include a high protein diet, alcohol and obesity. Aspirin is known to increase serum urate. Allopurinol can be used to reduce the level of urate in the circulation but it must not be commenced within 3 weeks of an acute attack as it can precipitate another incident.

73 h. This patient is suffering from arthritis mutilans – telescoping of the joints in her ring finger on her right hand. This arthritis is a form of psoriatic arthropathy, associated with the skin condition psoriasis. There are several similarities in this skin condition to rheumatoid arthritis. It is, therefore, important to consider psoriasis in any new patient presenting with rheumatoid features as the joint conditions may present before the skin lesions.

74 f. At the age of 16 years ankylosing spondylitis is 6 times more common in males than females. By the age of 30 it is twice as common in males. Typical presenting symptoms are morning back stiffness and progressive loss of spinal movement. Other features include hip and knee involvement and plantar fasciitis, as eluded to in this case study. Diagnosis is clinical but strongly supported by radiology, e.g. squaring of the vertebrae, formation of a 'bamboo spine' and obliteration of the sacroiliac joints. This is a rare example of a rheumatological condition being more common in males than females.

75 c. Osteoarthritis is the commonest joint condition; it is usually primary but

156

may be secondary to any joint disease or joint injury. Its mean age of onset is 50–60 years old. Pain is defined as being worse after periods of activity and towards the end of the day, with some eventual joint deformity and reduction of movements. Radiologically there are four main features; loss of joint space, subchondral sclerosis, cyst formation and marginal osteophytes. Treatment is mainly NSAIDs for pain relief and reduction of risk factors and exacerbating factors.

76 d. *Cryptosporidum parvum* is a protozoal infection that can cause a severe diarrhoea in immunocompromised individuals. Protozoal cysts adhere to the gut wall and cause a florid secretory diarrhoea that requires large volume fluid resuscitation. The organism can be found in cattle and can cause a self-limiting diarrhoea in immunocompetent individuals. Treatment is mainly supportiveas antibiotic therapy has not been proven to be effective.

77 e. *Cryptococcus neoformas* is a fungal infection usually associated with meningitis in HIV. The clinical signs may be masked by the damped immune response seen in immunocompromised individuals and thus the fever, neck stiffness and photophobia associated with inflammation of the meninges may be impaired or even lacking. *Cryptococcus* may be diagnosed by India Ink staining of a sample of CSF at lumbar puncture and carries a 20% mortality even with treatment.

78 b. Candidiasis is often seen in diabetics, those on immunosuppressive therapy and those with immunodeficiency. The most common manifestation is oral candidiasis with white plaques in the mouth and oropharynx. Oesophageal candidiasis presents with odynophagia (pain on swallowing – usually retrosternal) and dysphagia due to the pain. Treatment is usually with fluconazole or another associated 'azole' by mouth for a couple of weeks. Severe cases may merit using amphotericin with caution ('amphoterrible' – coined because of severe nephrotoxic side-effects).

79 c. Infection with the protozoan *Toxoplasma gondii* can cause encephalitis and cerebral abscesses of which the latter may catastrophically be misdiagnosed as primary cerebral tumour or stroke. The symptoms are those of a space-occupying lesion, may cause fitting, focal neurological deficit, confusion and personality change, and may be difficult to distinguish from a cerebrovascular event. MRI is the investigation of choice in imaging suspected toxoplasma infection and can prove to be spectacu-larly superior to CT scanning in defining numbers and character of lesions. Treatment with pyrimethamine in combinationwith sulfadiazine and folinic acid for at least 6 weeks can produce remarkable reversal of the clinical state.

80 a. Pneumocystis Jerovici pneumonia (formally called *Pneumocystis Carinii* Pneumonia (PCP)) is one of the most common life-threatening infections in HIV/AIDS. It

157

can act as a benchmark for the severity of immunosuppression as it is rarely seen with CD4 counts higher than 200/mm3. Prophylaxis when CD4 counts drop below 200/mm3 is given and co-trimoxazole (Trimethoprim and Sulfamethoxazole) is the agent of choice.

Chest signs may be clinically absent but the usual scenario is an HIV positive individual who is in frank respiratory compromise with hypoxia, tachypnoea, tachycardia with fine crepitations throughout the chest. Treatment is with high-dose

co-trimoxazole for up to 3 weeks with systemic corticosteroids for severe disease (defined as a PaO2 of less than 9.5kPa).

81 h. Lithium carbonate is a frequently used drug for both prophylaxis and treatment of mood disorders and has been termed a 'mood-stabiliser'. Classically used as a first-line agent in the long term treatment of bipolar disorder (manic-depression) it helps maintain euthymia and reduces up- and downswings of mood.

Side-effects of lithium can be severe and drug monitoring must be undertaken on a regular basis. Lithium toxicity can be precipitated by electrolyte derangements, most notably hyponatraemia, and may lead to nephrogenic diabetes insipidus characterised by an inability to concentrate water in the kidney and leading to dehydration and polydipsia that is resistant to desmopressin.

82 e. Eye movement desensitisation and reprocessing (EMDR) has been used with some success in those suffering from post-traumatic stress disorder (PTSD) following violent acts especially sexual abuse and trauma from combat. EMDR usually takes place over multiple sessions and involves the assessment of a patient for EMDR therapy including whether they are emotionally stable enough to start the process of therapy. Subsequent therapy sessions involve identifying a negative thought or image relating to the trauma and a positive thought or belief.

The remainder of the therapy involves uncoupling the negative thought process by typically following the therapists fingers across the visual field multiple times and to express the thought processes experienced at the time. Other modalities such as music or other tactile stimuli can be employed instead of eye movements. The aim of the process is to slowly replace the negative emotion experienced during sessions with the positive belief identified at the beginning of therapy. Closure of sessions involves written reflection of events between sessions and evaluation of the effectiveness of the self-calming measures.

Other modalities used in the treatment of PTSD involve the use of selective-serotonin reuptake inhibitors (SSRIs) and beta-blocking medication to reduce the symptoms of hyperarousal.

83 a. Schneider's first rank symptoms describe the spectrum of symptoms experienced by those with schizophrenia and are as follows:

1. Auditory hallucinations

2. Thought insertion

3. Thought withdrawal

4. Thought block

5. Thought broadcast

6. Somatic hallucinations

7. Lack of control over bodily function e.g. controlled by external forces

8. Delusions (fixed unshakeable beliefs)

Treatment involves the use of neuroleptics, either the older classes such as haloperidol or risperidone (with their risk of extra-pyramidal side-effects, e.g. parkinsonism and sedation profile) or the newer classes of neuroleptics such as olanzipine, clozap-ine and quetiapine. Haloperidol and risperidone are commonly used in the acute management of psychosis with the newer agents more useful for longer-term management. Clozapine must be monitored frequently for the serious side-effect of agranulocytosis; defined as a white blood cell count less than 500/mm3.

84 g. Anxiety attacks are often associated with situations such as speaking in public or being in a public place and share similar characteristics to the specific phobias. Agoraphobia (the fear of being in a public place) is one of the most commonly associated phobias with anxiety. Generalised anxiety disorders have no readily identifiable precipitant and anxiety attacks can occur daily over long periods of time. In this case the woman is exhibiting a panic disorder, manifest as anxiety when performing in public. There are many modalities used to counteract anxiety such as selective serotonin reuptake inhibitors, other classes of antidepressants and benzodiazepines (which should only be used as a last resort in intractable anxiety due to the dependence forming effects of benzodiazepines). Simple measures, however, are often overlooked and these include breathing exercises, dietary modifications including avoiding all caffeine-containing products and relaxation techniques. These should be at least considered as a first line before instituting medication, which may eventually become a long-term and unnecessary crutch.

85 d. Electroconvulsive therapy (ECT) is a highly effective form of treatment for severe depression that is refractive to medical therapy and especially useful in the treatment of depression associated with delusional symptoms. The process involves undergoing a short course of general anaesthesia with a muscle relaxant (to prevent muscle damage and rhabdomyolysis associated with rapid muscular contraction during the procedure) then passing of current via two electrodes across the brain. The effect is similar to a tonic–clonic seizure in both electrical brain activity and clinical effect with post-ictal amnesia and confusion being infrequent non-anaesthetic related side-effects. The reversal of mood is extremely rapid with the use of ECT and can produce profound effects in a short space of time making it an effective therapy for those at severe risk of self-harm or suicide in which antidepressant medication may take too long to have effect.

86 c. Gardeners expose themselves to many organisms if durable gloves are not worn and infections of the nailbed and surrounding area are common. These conditions are occasionally confused with fungal infections of the nailbed and scrapings for mycology can be taken if there is any doubt. Another common infection spread characteristically following rose-thorn pricks is with *Sporothrix* spp. This usually presents with characteristic tracks that spread distal to proximal.

87 b. Glomus tumour typically presents as a mass under the nail with severe pain as the most common feature. The bluish hue is another feature of this rare tumour that can resemble a subungval melanoma. Looking for other signs of melanoma can often be useful in differentiating between these two conditions.

88 e. Self-harm injuries commonly occur on the forearms and are more common in the female population. Injury to the radial and median nerves is most common in injuries to the wrist, the median nerve being especially vulnerable to slash injuries due to its relatively superficial course at the carpal tunnel. Radial nerve injury typically presents with an inability to extend the hand leading to wrist drop. The aide memoire 'BEST' (**b**ra-chioradialis, **e**xtensors of the forearm, **s**upinator and **t**riceps) describes the muscle of the forearm supplied by this nerve.

89 h. This injury is one of the most commonly injured bones of the carpal row, thought to be due to the higher stresses imposed on the scaphoid due to its unique position spanning both proximal and distal rows of the carpal bones. Falling on an outstretched hand is the mechanism of injury usually encountered in this type of injury, occasionally complicated by neurovascular compromise as with any fracture. Tenderness in the anatomical snuffbox forms a useful clinical reckoner if scaphoid fracture is suspected.

160

90 g. Associated with a diverse variety of conditions such as diabetes mellitus, acromegaly, rheumatoid arthritis and pregnancy, carpal tunnel syndrome (CTS) manifests with tingling and numbness that patients often describe as being relieved by shaking out their hands. Pain is typically complained of at night, and can be exacerbated by tapping over the carpal tunnel with the wrist extended (Tinel's test) or by stressing both wrists together into forced flexion (Phalen's test) and form a useful clinical screen for CTS. It is thought to be due to fluid retention in the case of pregnancy, diabetes and acromegaly although the exact mechanism is not known.

PAPER 2 ANSWERS

Answers and notes

Multiple choice questions (single best answer)

1 c. This patient needs to be admitted for an open reduction and internal fixation of the fracture. The key feature in this history is the rotation of the fragment. If the fracture was undisplaced and not rotated this could be managed in a backslab and followed up in fracture clinic however, since there is associated rotation the patient requires surgical management to achieve a successful outcome. On examination of this gentleman's hand it was noted that he was unable to form a fist due to swelling and pain (not uncommon with unrotated fractures either) but there was obvious rotation of his affected little finger.

2 c. The investigation most likely to be diagnostic is the MRI of the spine. Whilst the bone scan will be useful if the MRI scan does show metastases (which, in this case it did) alone it will not be diagnostic. Whilst it is important to exclude sinister causes of this gentleman's pain it is also important to exclude common causes of low back pain including discitis and disc prolapse, all of which may be identified on MRI or CT scan. This gentleman was found to have metastases in his spine and returned to a ter-tiary centre to have both chemotherapy and radiotherapy.

3 c. This case presents a difficult ethical dilemma that is not infrequently encountered and can require extremely sensitive handling of the situation. An adult that is unconscious or otherwise incompetent to make a decision with respect to understanding, weighing up the options and retaining information in order to make an informed decision about their medical care presents difficultly in deciding what is in the patient's best interest. A discussion with family members may sometimes help inform the decision; however, there is no legal requirement (for an otherwise competent adult) for assent from the family or close relatives before making decisions about medical care in situations where that adult cannot consent to treatment.

Refusing to perform surgery without blood is indeed a surgeon's prerogative as a splenectomy following trauma may be dangerous without the back-up of blood products and may ultimately cause more harm than good. However, this is not the right course of action as without surgery the prognosis is poor. Using crystalloid replacement is similarly not correct for the reasons above.

The brief clinical indicators point to a ruptured spleen in a hypotensive road traffic accident victim in whom delaying surgery any longer than is necessary would be seriously detrimental to the prognosis and would be labelled as medically unsafe.

Awaiting a court order in an emergency situation would take too long and would not allow the appropriate timely intervention (emergency surgery) to occur thus this should not be considered.

As the child is 14 years of age and a legal minor the parents have a legal right to dictate what medical treatment is appropriate for their child. However, in the case of emergency or life-threatening situations this may be overcome by the need to do what is in the patient's best interest. The four pillars of ethics are beneficence, non-maleficence, autonomy and justice, and should always be borne in mind when addressing ethical situations.

Applied to this case the surgeon would be covered from a legal and ethical standpoint to act in the patient's best interest and take the child to surgery, even if this is against the religious view of the parents. Further justification is that religious values of parents are not intrinsically inherent to children and should not be assumed to represent the true wishes of the child in a situation such as this. A sensible strategy would be to take the onus from the parents by stating that clinical need dictates this course of action and if there was any other way to proceed without transfusion it would have been explored. Often this abdicates the feeling of blame and responsibility that comes with making an active decision by taking the decision out of their hands.

4 c. Molluscum contagiosum is caused by a poxvirus and is most commonly seen in children. Lesions are typical in appearance and present as discrete papules sometimes with a surrounding area of mild erythema due to an eczematous process. A distinctive feature of molluscum contagiosum is the presence of a central core of keratin, which can be expressed from the lesions.

They are treated conservatively and will resolve on their own or can be squeezed between two fingernails to express the central keratin plug. Varicella zoster does give a similar picture;however, the absence of significant itch, blistering vesicles and distribution in a particular dermatome makes the diagnosis unlikely. Herpes simplex is found in two subtypes: HSV 1 affecting the oral and buccal mucosa causing 'cold sores' and HSV 2 affecting primarily the genital tract (although both types can be found almost anywhere in the body). The lesions are transmissible through direct contact, e.g. kissing, and may be painful and ulcerated with small eruptive vesicles. The lesions will settle spontaneously although in the immunocompromised or elderly a prolonged

163

course may occur. Eczema presents as an itchy rash with typical erythema and excoriation of the

skin from scratching. Lesions are neither papular nor discrete entities and characteristically affect flexor surfaces. Pityriasis versicolor is a skin condition affecting primarily young adults and is due to *Malassezia* yeasts, a normal skin commensal. Areas of macular hypopigmentation are seen in persons of dark skin colour with a faint brownish colour in those persons of light skin colour. Microscopic examination of skin scrapings reveals the yeasts clumped in short balls and longer hyphae.

5 d. Arthropathy is a condition that is usually associated with psoriasis and may in fact sometimes be the first presentation of psoriasis in a patient with no obvious skin lesions. The arthropathy can mimic many other rheumatological conditions including rheumatoid arthritis and osteoarthritis, however, usually presents in one of four patterns:

1. Distal interphalangeal joint involvement.

2. Rheumatoid-like joint changes.

3. Large joint involvement.

4. Seronegative-type joint changes.

Up to 10% of psoriatics will suffer with some kind of joint change associated with skin disease. Eczema can be broadly classified into exogenous, i.e. usually due to an allergic or irritant stimulus, and endogenous, i.e. no identifiable precipitant.

The latter classification further subdivides into atopic eczema, eczema associated with venous insufficiency, eczema affecting the sebaceous glands, discoid eczema and asteatotic eczema,

which tends to affect the elderly (especially those who are subject to hospital and nursing home washing and bathing).

Eczema responds to emollients to keep the skin from drying and atopic eczema usually benefits from topical steroid cream.

Secondary bacterial infection can manifest in broken eczematous skin and a topical steroid and antibacterial combination therapy or even systemic antibiotics may be employed to both eradicate the infection and return the skin to a more balanced level of hydration.

6 d. This investigation is useful in the screening for two common urological conditions: prostate cancer and benign prostatic hyperplasia (BPH). Epidemiological evidence suggests BPH is more common in the Afro-Caribbean population and may be

linked to higher testosterone levels. Suprapubic catheterisation is a useful therapeutic and diagnostic procedure for those whose urethral catheterisation is contraindicated, such as urethral stricture or pelvic trauma where there is a risk of urethral rupture. In an elderly gentleman presenting with such symptoms, it is usually advisable to perform a digital rectal examination, prostate-specific antigen, renal function and urinalysis as part of routine management.

7 e. The condition described is typical of retroperitoneal fibrosis (peri-aortitis). It is an autoimmune condition where there is progressive fibrosis surrounding the aorta, into which the ureters become embedded causing renal obstruction, failure and retention. Methysergide has a particular association and may still be seen in use for resistant migraine. Paracetamol can lead to acute tubular necrosis as an adverse side-effect and acyclovir may cause crystal deposition in cases of dehydration. Gold injections should also be monitored regularly for renal side-effects by follow-up urinalysis for proteinuria. Rosiglitazone must be used with caution in patients with pre-existing renal impairment but itself has few renal side-effects in normal kidneys.

8 d. This lady is suffering an allergic reaction to the antibiotics.

Despite having had five previous doses and no known drug allergies these symptoms of facial flushing and tingling in her hands are characteristic of an allergic reaction. More severe cases of allergy/anaphylaxis may result in shortness of breath and chest pain. Although this was not the case here, these should always be noted as important negatives in the patients notes. It is important to stop all antibiotics in this case to assess the response to steroids and antihistamines as there may be another underlying cause for these symptoms and failure to identify this could lead to malpractice cases.

9 a. This lady needs to continue rehabilitation before being discharged home. Being a recurrent attender should pose the question of whether there is an underlying social issue. This lady, although medically fit, would not benefit from being immediately discharged under GP care as this option has been available to her but she has repeatedly chosen to call an ambulance.

Remaining in hospital until she feels ready to leave would lead to a number of problems both financially and physically in terms of acquiring hospital infections and taking up an acute bed. Being assessed by social services is a realistic option, although in reality this takes time and means an extended stay in hospital whilst the process is completed. Placement in a local cottage hospital is a good compromise; it allows continued rehabilitation with physiotherapists whilst being less at risk of developing further infections.

10 b. Signs of an ischaemic limb include the **6 P's**:

• **P**allor

• **P**ulseless

• **P**araesthesiae

• **P**ainful

• **P**aralysis

• **P**erishingly cold

From the history we know that this lady is suffering from the pallor and pulselessness described above. She has a present femoral pulse but not below that level which suggests an embolus at the mid-femoral level. The symptoms are not indicative of arterial insufficiency and there has been no mention of an abdominal mass to suggest an abdominal arterial aneurysm. In cases of venous ulceration you would expect to see changes in the skin, including breakdown of the epidermal level which is not described here.

Potential sources of emboli in this case include the left atrium, heart valves and from the aorta among others.

This lady went on to have an embolectomy and post-operative management with unfractionated heparin. Unfortunately due to her age and her concomitant chest problems her outcome was not as good as desired and she died 36 hours post-operatively.

11 e. Panic disorders are seen 2 to 3 times more commonly in females than males and are diagnosed according to strict criteria involving sensations of choking, tingling or numbness, chest tightness and shortness of breath, fear of losing control and a variety of other perceived symptoms. In addition to the presence of these symptoms a diagnosis of panic disorder is only valid if there is an additional persistent worry for a period greater than 1 month about recurrence of attacks, the consequences of having another attack and a significant behavioural modification as a result of a panic attack, e.g. avoiding public places. Panic disorders exhibit a bimodal distribution in prevalence with peaks seen in late adolescence and then again in the mid-30s.

There have been a wide variety of medical co-morbiditiesassociated with panic disorders: irritable bowel syndrome, COPD,cardiomyopathy, hypertension, migraine headache, mitral valve prolapse to name a few of the more studied examples. Agoraphobia is often seen with panic disorder and is estimated to be present in between 30% and 50% of cases of diagnosed panic disorder.

Treatment modalities used for panic disorder include cognitive behavioural therapy involving exposure and subsequent desensitisation to panic-inducing stimuli, respiratory training to help break the cycle of reinforcement of panic-induced hyperventilation and medical therapy usually in the form of antidepressant medication with selective serotonin reuptake inhibitors as first-line followed by tricyclic antidepressants as a second-line modality.

12 c. PTSD is defined as a pathological anxiety reaction that develops following an extreme traumatic stressor (often an act of physical violence) witnessed or experienced by an individual.

Features manifest as mood disturbance, a re-experiencing of the event, hypervigilance (exaggerated startle reaction) and avoidance of stimuli (e.g. location) associated with the event. It is differentiated from the very similar condition of acute stress disorder by the duration of symptoms. PTSD symptoms usuallyoccur a few months from the sentinel event and can last for anywhere between less than 3 months to greater than 6 months. Acute stress disorders typically occur within 1 month of a traumatic event and last for less than 1 month from onset.

Depressive symptoms make a diagnosis of depression a differential to consider; however, there are only a few of the symptoms of a depressive episode listed in the clinical vignette and the addition of nightmares associated with a history of a traumatic event alongside the features of a pathologically heightened sense of awareness (hypervigilance and exaggerated startle response) make this diagnosis unlikely.

Schizoid personality disorders present with behavioural manifestations that are typically detached from close relationships, aloof and exhibiting signs of anhedonia (inability to enjoy oneself).

167

Rarely seen in the clinical setting this diagnosis forms part of the Cluster A (odd, eccentric) classification of personality disorders along with schizotypal and paranoid personality disorders.

GAD describes a chronic anxiety state characterised by disproportional worry about a wide range of life events that cause impairment to normal social functioning. The pertinent features associated with GAD are of anxiety that occurs for most days for greater than 6 months and manifest with greater than three somatic symptoms such as sleep disturbance, poor concentration and mood disturbance.

13 b. This clinical picture represents acute lymphocytic leukaemia.

The child is in the right age category, approximately 4–8 years of age. Symptoms of this condition may be split into bone marrow failure, systemic symptoms and local symptoms. Systemic symptoms include malaise and weight loss with sweats or anorexia being the most common. Acute myeloid leukaemia commonly presents in the elderly approximately aged 70 years old.

A chest X-ray may be helpful in the diagnosis, a mediastinal mass is occasionally seen. For confirmation of the diagnosis a trephine bone marrow biopsy is required.

14 c. It is chronic myeloid leukaemia that involves the translocation of the so-called Philadelphia chromosome.

15 a. Hodgkin's lymphoma typically presents with a picture of painless localised lymphadenopathy with systemic features associated with malignancy of weight loss, fevers, night sweats and lethargy. Often seen in young men around the age of

20 years there is a second peak in middle age. Almost pathognomonic of Hodgkin's lymphoma is the interesting association of pain upon drinking alcohol and this sometimes may be the primary complaint of those presenting with the disease. The pathological hallmark of Hodgkin's lymphoma is the Reed Sternberg cell, sometimes referred to as owl's eyes.

Infectious mononucleosis is caused by the Epstein–Barr virus and commonly presents insidiously with fatigue and malaise with a sore throat being the second most common symptom.

Penicillin derivatives such as amoxicillin should be avoided in the treatment of infectious mononucleosis as they may cause a maculopapular rash.

Non-Hodgkin's lymphoma is typically classified into low grade, intermediate-grade and high-grade depending on the clinical behaviour of the tumour. Presenting

168

most often with peripheral lymphadenopathy there may be involvement of bone marrow causing abnormal blood counts and constitutional features of cancer are common reported symptoms.

Polycythaemia rubra vera is a disorder affecting the totipotent haematopoeitic stem cells and causes a varying degree of overproduction of erythrocytes, leucocytes and platelets. Often causing vascular thromboses patients may present with stroke, myocardial infarction, deep vein thromboses or pulmonary emboli. Arterial thromboses are, interestingly, seen 3 times more commonly than venous thromboses.

MDS actually describes a group of haematopoeitic disorders that many authors group as a form of pre-malignancy.

Characterised by either a hypercellular or hypocellular bone marrow with abnormal forms seen on peripheral blood smear this disorder is likely underestimated in the population over 70 and may be increasing in incidence due to the relative increase in blood tests taken on arrival to hospital as compared to years ago. Clinically the symptoms of anaemia or thrombocytopaenia may be the only clues to an abnormal marrow and is often the mode of diagnosis in the majority of elderly patients presenting to hospital with nebulous constitutional upset.

16 b.   The symptoms and biochemical markers of renal failure and lung involvement, i.e. haemoptysis should raise the concern of hepatopulmonary diseases such as Goodpasture's syndrome. A proliferative glomerulonephritis associated with pulmonary infiltrates causing haemoptysis (sometimes massive in nature) are the pathological hallmarks of this aggressive disease. Antibodies to basement membranes affecting both glomeruli and alveoli are the typical antibodies exhibited by patients with Goodpasture's syndrome. Anti-neutrophil cytoplasmic antibodies (ANCA) are more strongly associated with systemic vasculitides such as Wegener's granulomatosis (PR3-ANCA), microscopic polyangiitis and Churg–Strauss disease (MPO-ANCA). Anti-SCL 70 is classically associated with systemic sclerosis, anti-mitochondrial antibodies often seen in cirrhosis of liver and biliary tree and rheumatoid factor associated with rheumatoid disease and associated syndromes, e.g. Felty's syndrome. It is worth noting, however, that no antibody is entirely specific or sensitive to a particular disease and there are many patients without any disease who will exhibit positive antibody titres.

17 e.   Carpal tunnel syndrome (CTS) is commonly associated with rheumatoid arthritis but lesser known but important other associations include dialysis, pregnancy, diabetes mellitus and hypothyroidism. Symptoms are always in the distribution of the median nerve and are characteristically described by patients to affect them at night, relieved by shaking the hands out and the symptoms of which can be often brought on in clinic by Tinel's test (tapping over the extended wrist) and less reliably by Phalen's test (forced flexion at the wrist). Treatment options in chronological order of trial should include wrist splinting, local steroid injection (symptomatic relief only) then consideration of surgical decompression of the carpal tunnel indicated in cases of (a) prolonged symptoms and (b) neurological symptoms, e.g. thenar eminence wasting. Plain radiographs of the wrist and hand are unlikely to be of any use in the management of CTS, however, may provide useful baseline views for assessing radiographic progression of rheumatoid disease.

18 d. Investigation of breast lumps involves triple assessment. The gold standard for this varies in accordance with the age of the patients.

All patients require:

• Clinical assessment.

• Imaging (either mammogram or ultrasound).

• Cytology/histology.

The imaging is dependent on the patient's age. For patients under the age of 35 years old an ultrasound is the most appropriate form of imaging due to the ductal and dense nature of the breast tissue. After the age of 35 years, breast tissue becomes increasingly fatty which is better imaged with mammography. In patients with breast implants it may be necessary to consider CT scanning.

19 c. There is radiological evidence of an abscess which will require drainage. In the first instance a needle aspiration under local anaesthetic is the most appropriate treatment. In the event that this is unsuccessful due to the pus being too thick or not achieving symptomatic relief an incision and drainage should be considered. This treatment should always be followed up with a course of antibiotics, usually flucloxacillin or erythromycin if penicillin allergic. Patients should be advised to continue to breastfeed. Although this may provide discomfort it will aid the healing process and in addition it is safe to do so whilst being on antibiotics. In all cases pus should be sent off to exclude an inflammatory carcinoma.

20 c. Marfan's syndrome is an inherited connective tissue disorder that affects the expression of the fibrillin gene leading to defects in the connective tissue of the ocular, skeletal and cardiovascular system. Mitral valve prolapse, tall, spindly stature, ectopia lentis (lens dislocation) as well as aortic involvement such as aortic-root dilatation, aortic regurgitation and aortic dissection are associated with the syndrome. William's syndrome is a neu-rodevelopmental disorder with cardiovascular abnormalities and typical facial appearances. Hypercalcaemia is also commonly seen. Most importantly in this syndrome is the association of supravalvular aortic outflow obstruction, which may be severe enough to cause sudden death. Down's syndrome is a disorder of mental development, behaviour and associated with characteristic features including a single palmar crease, upslant-ing palpebral fissure and a flat nasal bridge. Ocular involvementis legion ranging from refractive errors as the most common to congenital cataracts. Lens dislocation, however, is a relatively rare event. Turner's syndrome is a disease affecting females and presents with short stature and signs of ovarian dysfunction.

Widely spaced nipples and a webbed neck are often quoted features of this disease and genetic analysis reveals a 45 XO karyotype. Reiter's syndrome is a rheumatological manifestation of the triad of conjunctivitis, urethritis and arthritis, and classically occurs following a sexually-transmitted infection although this can be seen after a bout of infectious diarrhoea. It is a seronegative arthropathy, so-called because rheumatoid factor is negative in these patients and is grouped with reactive arthropathy, enteropathy-associated arthropathy and ankylosing spondylitis.

21 d. Sjögren's syndrome (keratoconjunctivitis sicca) manifests as dryness of the mucous membranes leading to dry eyes, dry mouth (xerostomia) and occasionally dryness of the tracheobronchial tree. Investigations include the Schirmer test, which assesses the amount of tear production from the eye with a reduction to less than 5mm of tearing after 5 minutes on a strip of filter paper suggestive of the condition. Erythrocyte sedimentation rate and autoantibodies, especially anti-Ro and anti-La (SS-A and SS-B) are frequently raised in Sjögren's syndrome.

Anterior uveitis is associated with the seronegative arthropathies, a group of arthritic conditions so-called because they do not exhibit a positive rheumatoid factor. Classified into enteropathy-associated arthritis, reactive arthritis (including Reiter's syndrome), psoriatic arthritis and ankylosing spondylitis are commonly associated with extra-articular features such as inflammation of the (anterior) uveal tract comprising iris, ciliary body and choroid. Symptoms of anterior uveitis include pain in the affected eye, tear production, blurred vision and occasionally photophobia. Acute glaucoma can present in a similar fashion to anterior uveitis and must be differentiated if appropriate treatment can be instituted. One of the true ocular emergencies it presents with an acutely painful, red eye with both conjunctival and ciliary vessel injection. The pupil is fixed, dilated and oval in shape and the intraocular pressure is high. Beta-blockade, acetazolamide and topical steroids form the mainstay of treatment. Subconjunctival haemorrhage presents with an acute red eye consisting of bright red sclera with a rim around the limbus.

The pupil is normal, which allows differentiation from the other causes of red eye. Retinal vein occlusion commonly occurs in elderly hypertensive patients and presents with an acute deterioration in visual acuity. It can be detected on fundoscopy as

either a wedge deficit on the retina (due to a branch retinal vein occlusion) or when central presents with dot and blot haemorrhages or florid retinal haemorrhages leading to the description of the appearance as a 'stormy sunset'. Photocoagulation is the treatment of choice in preventing the neovascular complications of retinal vein occlusion; however, no medical therapy has been demonstrated to be curative once the event has occurred.

22 e. Cushing's disease is associated with hyperglycaemia due to the glucocorticoid effect of cortisol and associated steroids.

Cushing's disease describes a specific disease of hypercortisolae-mia due to excess ACTH from a pituitary tumour. It is a subdivision of Cushing's syndrome, which describes glucocorticoid excess usually due to excess ACTH (90%) of which the majority (90%) are due to ACTH-producing pituitary tumours. Other causes of excess ACTH leading to Cushing's syndrome include ectopic production from certain lung and carcinoid tumours and rarely over-administration of ACTH. Primary causes of Cushing's syndrome include steroid use, adrenal tumours and alcohol abuse. Addison's disease can be thought simplistically as the opposite of Cushing's syndrome as primary adrenal failure leads to low levels of circulating corticosteroids. Thus hypoglycaemia, hypotension and hyperkalaemia and hyponatraemia occur. Liver failure tends to present with hypoglycaemia due to impaired liver function leading to poor glycogen production (resulting in low 'glucose' stores during periods of fasting) and impaired fatty acid metabolism. Insulinomas are classically associated with severe hypoglycaemia due to excess production of insulin and may be biochemically tested for by assay of c-peptide levels (which are cleaved from insulin precursors to release physiologically active insulin). In cases where exogenous insulin may be abused thus mimicking the effects of insulinoma, c-peptide levels can be taken; they will be high in insulinoma and within normal limits or low in exogenous insulin administration (as c-peptide is not present in synthetic insulin). Gliclazide is a sulphonylurea that is similar in structure to sulpha antibiotics. The mechanism of action as a hypoglycaemic agent was discovered when malnourished and starved patients were given sulpha antibiotics leading to hypoglycaemic attacks and acts by increasing endogenous insulin production (sulphonylureas squeeze the pancreas!). Sulphonylureas should be used with caution in the elderly because of the decreased awareness for hypoglycaemic attacks and thus inability to counteract the effects (e.g. by taking sweet foods/drinks). The duration of action of the sulphonylureas is long and therefore any diabetic presenting to hospital with hypoglycaemia on sulphonylurea tablets must be either admitted for blood glucose observation for a 24-hour period until the effect has worn off or in exceptional circumstances where they themselves or those around them are able to measure the blood glucose and know how to counteract any hypoglycaemia, may be allowed

to return home but with a low threshold to return to hospital if there is any doubt about the effectiveness of treatment.

23 c. Clues from the vignette include the fact that the patient is asking for other therapeutic options other than tablets and the fact that the T4 level is elevated in the face of a high thyroid-stimulating hormone (TSH), which in the absence of a secondary cause for hyperthyroidism (e.g. hypothalamic or pituitary disease producing high TSH) is discordant with the clinical state. The most likely explanation is chronic under-treatment of hypothyroidism leading to a raised TSH as the pituitary tries to compensate for low levels of T4 followed by over-replacement prior to the clinic appointment in order to try to give the biochemical appearance of compliance.

Subclinical hypothyroidism presents with a T4 that is in the normal range but at the low end of the spectrum with a raised TSH. Treatment of subclinical hypothyroidism depends on the clinical state and often these patients are followed up with regular interval blood tests to assess the need for thyroxine replacement. Sick euthyroid syndrome is often seen biochemically as a low TSH and low T4 (and T3) and occurs in the absence of any pre-existing thyroid or hypothalamo-pituitary disease. It can occur for a number of reasons including gastrointestinal and cardiovascular disease and is defined from intrinsic thyroid dysfunction by the resolution of abnormal thyroid tests with resolution of the underlying non-thyroid illness. Inadequate replacement with thyroxine would lead to a low T4 and a high TSH (simply slightly 'milder' biochemical indices of hypothyroidism than frank untreated hypothyroidism) and the opposite would lead to high T4 associated with a depressed TSH (by the negative feedback mechanism).

24 e. Whilst all of the options are correct, the most important is to complete a primary survey. Once this has been done the full extent of the situation will become clear and it will then be more appropriate to ask for help and order further investigations.

25 e. Erythema nodosum has no association with infective endocarditis. Retinal haemorrhages are seen in the form of Roth spots. Vasculitis accounts for Osler's nodes, splinter haemorrhages, Roth spots and Janeway lesions.

26 b. Furosemide is a loop diuretic. When given i.v. furosemide can reduce arteriolar vasodilatation which is a beneficial action independent to their diuretic effect. ACE inhibitors have an adjunct affect when used in combination with diuretics but in this situation optimisation of the diuretic therapy is the first step in management of this patient. Whilst bumetanide is a useful drug it is a loop diuretic and there is limited benefit of adding this into his treatment regime. Metolazone is a thiazide diuretic and is known to cause a profound diuresis. It has a role in severe hear failure resistant to large doses of loop diuretics.

27 b. Cocaine is known to cause spasm of coronary arteries and its abuse should always be suspected in cardiac sounding chest pain in a young person. Amphetamines are also known to cause cardiac arrhythmias.

28 d. This case is describing Marfan's syndrome. It is associated with mitral valve prolapse and a dilated aortic root. The prolapse gives a mid-systolic click followed by a systolic murmur heard at the apex. Associations of Marfan's syndrome also include lens detachment and a marfarnoid habitus where arm span is characteristically longer than height.

29 b. Serum potassium is important to monitor in patients on digoxin as hypokalaemia can potentiate the effects of digoxin leading to toxicity.

30 c. Ibuprofen and other non-steroidal anti-inflammatory drugs (NSAIDs) should be avoided if possible in anything other than mild renal failure (arbitrarily defined as a glomerular filtration rate of between 20 and 50mL/minute). The mechanism of

action of the NSAIDS is to inhibit cyclo-oxygenase enzymes thus decreasing the amount of prostaglandin production (PGE2 and PGI2 especially). Prostaglandins are involved in the inflammatory cascade but additionally have effect on the maintenance of renal blood flow, especially at the site of the glomerular afferent arterioles. Thus the decrease in production of prostaglandins in patients who are susceptible to changes in renal homeostasis (such as those with renal impairment) can cause decompensation of function. Alternative analgesic modalities should be sought that can safely be used in patients with suboptimal renal function.

31 b. Post-streptococcal glomerulonephritis is associated with streptococcal upper respiratory tract infections and usually presents anywhere between a week and 3 weeks post-infection.

Haematuria, often described as dark or smoky rather than frank blood, is frequently encountered. Oedema, especially of the peri-orbital region, is a common presentation in children with post-streptococcal glomerulonephritis and accompanies proteinuria, hypertension and oliguria. Treatment is usually supportive with spontaneous resolution being the rule. Minimal change glomerulonephritis is the most common cause of the nephritic syndrome in children. Symptoms are similar with oedema, hypertension and association with upper respiratory tract infection; however, thromboembolic events due to loss of anti-clotting products in the urine make the diagnosis more likely. Corticosteroids form the mainstay of treatment. Henoch–Schönlein purpura is a vasculitis of small vessels that affects young males twice as frequently as females and manifests as punctate bleeding points associated with abdominal pain and gastrointestinal bleeding.

Characteristic 'bruising' occurs over the buttocks and lower limbs and may sometimes be mistaken for non-accidental injury in a child. Berger's disease is the commonest primary glomerulonephritis worldwide. Immune complex deposition is thought to be part of the pathophysiology of Berger's disease with ensuing glomerular damage and renal failure. Treatment may be supportive only if the degree of renal failure is mild. Rapidly progressive glomerulonephritis describes a pathological reduction in glomerular filtration rate over a short space of time and may be associated with anti-glomerular basement membrane antibodies, immune complex deposition or vasculitis-associated disease.

Immunosuppression is the treatment modality of choice.

32 d. Hyperkalaemia is associated with CRF and is most important in the setting of acute on when levels can be rapidly elevated due to a sharp fall in glomerular filtration rate CRF. Treatment of acute severe hyperkalaemia (potassium level above 6.5mmol/L or electrocardiogram changes) is managed firstly by intravenous injection of 10mL of 10% calcium gluconate as cardioprotection. Secondly infusion of e.g. 10 units of short-acting insulin with 50mL of 50% dextrose over 30 minutes will shift potassium intracellularly. Correcting the underlying cause, e.g. hypovolaemia may stabilise the potassium level, however, depletion of total body stores of potassium may be indicated and can be achieved by using calcium resonium. Other electrolyte abnormalities may be a dilutional hyponatraemia secondary to fluid retention, hyperphosphataemia and associated hypocalcaemia due to reduced renal hydroxylation of vitamin D with uraemia and metabolic acidosis due to impaired hydrogen ion excretion.

Neurological manifestations of CRF include restless legs syndrome, peripheral neuropathy and non-specific signs such as dizziness and headache associated with dialysis.

33 c. Frusemide is an example of a loop diuretic and has action at the loop of Henlé. Other loop diuretics include ethacrynic acid and bumetanide. The mechanism of action is one of inhibition of the sodium/potassium/chloride co-transporter in the thick ascending limb of the loop of Henlé and inhibits reabsorption of the above electrolytes at this site. Renal losses of sodium of up to 15–20% are seen causing a loss of concentrating power at the loop and thus loss of free water. Acetazolamide is a carbonic-anhydrase inhibitor acting at the proximal convoluted tubule causing increased excretion of sodium bicarbonate with resultant loss of sodium, potassium and free water. The effect is self-limiting as levels of bicarbonate fall thus producing a temporary diuresis. Osmotic agents are not commonly used in the treatment of fluid overload and are more useful in the management of raised intracranial pressure; however, mannitol is an example of an osmotic agent that acts on the parts of the nephron freely permeable to water (proximal convoluted tubule, descending limb of the loop and collecting tubule). Water is drawn into the tubular lumen by osmosis with relatively marginal effect on sodium loss from the kidney. Thiazide drugs such as bendrofluazide and the newer agent indapamide act at the distal convoluted tubule to reduce sodium and chloride reabsorption. Potassium loss is significant with the thiazide diuretics and is due to a relative increase in the electrolyte gradient in the collecting duct essentially flushing away potassium. Spironolactone, amiloride and triamterene are examples of potassium-sparing diuretics with spirono-lactone being especially useful in conditions of hyperaldo-steronism such as Conn's disease (primary aldosteronism) and hepatic cirrhosis.

34 b. Oliguria is not an indication for dialysis itself and the cause should be investigated and treated, e.g. hypovolaemia.

Manifestations of oliguria such as fluid overload refractory to treatment or build-up of toxins such as urea and nitrogenous compounds may, however, influence the decision to dialyse.

A useful mnemonic for remembering the indications for dialysis is 'AEIOU' standing for Acidosis, Electrolyte abnormalities, Ingestions, Overload and Uraemic symptoms. Severe or worsening metabolic acidosis with a pH ↕ 7.2 and persistent hyperkalaemia ☐7mmol/L are good markers of the need for dialysis.

Fluid overload, e.g. pulmonary oedema, that is likely to cause respiratory embarrassment and/or cardiovascular instabilit may be adequately managed with dialysis when medical therapy has failed. In the setting of acute overdose, especially with metabolic derangement as may be seen with aspirin overdose, dialysis can be a useful means of stabilising a patient until adequate acid–base homeostasis is achieved.

35 c. In early disease there are no clinical findings. With disease progression myoclonus and gait disorder may be seen but very unlikely to be present at the onset of the condition. A CT scan of the brain may show diffuse cortical atrophy in late disease but again in early disease there are often no radiological signs.

Two of the commonest features to develop are memory impairment and language dysfunction, and dominant inheritance is seen in some families with an approximate age of onset of 50–60 years. Whilst insight remains depression is a common feature. As the disease progresses and insight is lost depression understandably becomes a less common feature.

36 c. In a case such as this one a diagnosis of a subarachnoid haemorrhage needs to be excluded. From the history it sounds as though the patient is quite well but she is describing the characteristic history of the worst pain ever experienced with no exacerbating or relieving factors. Subarachnoid haemorrhage can be fatal if it is not diagnosed and discussed with the neurosurgical team promptly. In many cases it can lead to fluctuations in the Glasgow Coma Scale requiring intensive monitoring and nursing. Whilst meningitis is important to rule out, the history is not classical for this. Subdural haemorrhages are most commonly seen in the elderly or in those patients who abuse alcohol. Benign intracranial pressure is most commonly seen in younger patients (20–40 years), usually females, particularly those with a raised body mass index.

37 d. *Bacillus cereus* is often associated with refried rice and is the culprit behind diarrhoea and vomiting that occurs soon after ingestion of food colonised by the bacterium. A mnemonic to help remember the association between *B. cereus* and rice is 'Eat refried rice? Be serious!' The onset of symptoms can be very rapid, anywhere between 1 and 5 hours from ingestion.

Clostridium botulinum can be found in many processed foods and has been associated with 'floppy baby syndrome'. This is due to the release of botulinum toxin usually associated with babies who have been fed honey and subsequently suffer vomiting and even paralysis. Rotavirus is another important cause of diarrhoea in children and is often responsible for outbreaks of playground diarrhoea. It is self-limiting and will resolve with adequate fluid rehydration and rest. *Cryptosporidium parvum* is a fungal infection commonly associated with HIV infection and usually resolves unless the patient is severely immunocompromised, i.e. CD4 count ⬇ 200. Treatment is supportive as there are no effective antimicrobial agents of proven value. *Escherichia coli* is possibly one of the more notorious causes of infective diarrhoea and has many subtypes. Enterotoxic *E. coli* is frequently associated with travel to different climates and cultures and has been aptly named 'traveller's diarrhoea'. As with almost

177

all the types of diarrhoea the treatment is fluid rehydration. Antibiotics are not used unless there are signs of systemic compromise.

38 e. Budd–Chiari syndrome is due to obstruction of the hepatic vein causing back-pressure and eventual damage to the liver.

Approximately one-third of cases have no identifiable cause; however, associations between hypercoagulable states have been well described in the literature. Oral contraceptive pill, polycythaemia rubra vera as well as haematological and intra-abdominal malignancy may all predispose to this catastrophic syndrome. Diagnosis is usually by venous phase CT scan, which delineates the filling defect in the hepatic vein and even inferior vena cava. Ultrasound of the liver may be a useful non-invasive bedside investigation to demonstrate retrograde flow in the portal system due to outflow obstruction and hence strengthen the diagnosis. Viral hepatitis may present similarly but usually with jaundice and right upper quadrant pain with or without a palpable liver. Gross ascites and signs of portal hypertension are not usually manifest without chronic liver disease and this goes against an acute infectious cause. Epstein–Barr virus infection can cause hepatomegaly and may occur post infectious mononucleosis but similarly to viral hepatitis does not usually cause a picture of chronic liver disease. Wilson's disease is a rare inherited disorder of copper metabolism causing hepatolenticular degeneration and deposition of copper in liver and basal ganglia.

It causes both movement disorders and liver failure in those not identified and treated early. Deposition of copper in Descemet's membrane in the eye causing Kayser–Fleischer rings is pathognomonic of this disease. α1-antitrypsin deficiency affects both lungs and liver causing emphysema and chronic liver disease. α1-antitrypsin is a protease involved in damping down inflammatory cascades and plays an especially important role in the protection of alveoli from protease damage in the lungs. It is associated with chronic liver disease and hepatocellular carcinoma in adults in approximately one-fourth of all α1-antitrypsin deficient patients.

39 c. This man is suffering from Crohn's disease (CD). The combination of clinical pattern and colonscopic appearance makes the diagnosis unlikely to be ulcerative or other types of colitis.

Aphthous ulceration is often one of the earliest signs on colons-copy and occur anywhere from mouth to anus thus differentiating CD from ulcerative colitis (UC), which occurs proximally from the rectum occasionally involving the terminal ileum (backwash ileitis). CD can be thought of as a transmural inflammatory process with multiple skip lesions associated with a cobblestone pattern. The mnemonic, 'a thick old

Crone skipping down a cobblestone pavement', sums up the histological and colonscopic appearance of CD neatly. Anal and perianal diseases are also a hallmark of CD very rarely seen in UC; this man is likely complaining of an anal fissure causing severe pain on passing stool and thus strengthens the diagnosis. Barium follow-throughis an extremely useful investigation in eliciting small bowel involvement of disease and the pathological hallmark of small bowel CD of rose-thorn-type ulceration may be seen.

40 b. A typical regimen for the management of diabetic ketoacidosis (DKA) is outlined below:

1. Start an infusion of 50 units of short-acting insulin in 50 mL of 0.9% sodium chloride at a high rate (e.g. 6 units/hour) with 5 L fluid replacement with 0.9% sodium chloride.

2. Once blood glucose levels are below 15 mmol/L convert to 5% dextrose fluid replacement and halve infusion rate (e.g. 3 units/hour).

3. Monitor urine for ketones and once ketones are negative or very low and the patient is eating and drinking normally stop the insulin infusion.

4. If the patient is not eating normally convert insulin infusion to sliding scale with hourly blood glucose measurement.

5. Potassium is driven into cells by insulin and will thus appear initially high due to lack of insulin but will rapidly drop with sliding scale. Titrate up to 40 mmol/hour against the serum potassium.

The rationale for large volume fluid rehydration is that high levels of blood glucose cause a massive osmotic diuresis and may be associated with vomiting. Fluid losses through the kidneys and gastrointestinal tract lead to serious dehydration. High levels of insulin infusion are used to suppress ongoing ketogenesis, which will happen hours after the blood glucose levels have been brought down and thus urinary monitoring of ketones is vital to guide requirements to sliding scale. Metabolic acidosis will respond to fluid rehydration and will correct with the breakdown of ketone bodies, a byproduct of free fatty acid metabolism. Type I diabetics eating and drinking normally should be given subcutaneous insulin 30 minutes pre-prandially with insulin infusion stopped 1 hour after the meal to ensure adequate insulin cover during the transition. Basal bolus insulin or intermediate-acting insulin will not be adequate to suppress ketogenesis, which is key in correcting the metabolic acidosis and thus should not be used in the acute management of DKA.

41 d. This woman is exhibiting the symptoms and signs of diverticulitis. Left iliac fossa pain associated with a high white cell count, raised inflammatory markers and constitutional upset makes the diagnosis likely. A tender palpable mass in the abdomen is occasionally found on clinical examination but is not an indication for surgery as many can be managed conservatively with antibiotics such as cefuroxime and metronidazole. If an abscess is suspected that is resilient to medical therapy, CT-guided percutaneous drainage is a relatively safe and feasible option. CT scanning of the abdomen is a very useful imaging modality that carries none of the complications, e.g. perforation that direct visualisation of the bowel does. Recent trials of risk factors for diverticular perforation have identified a possible role for opioid and non-steroidal anti-inflammatory drug (NSAID) analgesia in the development of such complications. Long-term use of opioid analgesia has been shown to increase intracolonic pressure and hence possibly increase the risk of mechanical perforation of diverticu-lae. NSAIDs have been linked to an alteration in mucosal blood flow via prostaglandin inhibition leading to a consistentlyidentified risk of perforation in up to 20% of diverticular complications. This should, however, not preclude the use of NSAIDs but guide sensible prescribing of this often feared analgesic agent.

42 d. Normal portal venous pressure is between 8 and 15 cmH2O. Portal hypertension occurs when there is outflow obstruction to the portal system and can be evidenced by clinical manifestations and ultrasonographically, with reversal of flow along the portal vein. Obstruction can be classified as pre-hepatic, (e.g.portal vein thrombosis secondary to neonatal umbilical infection), hepatic (e.g. cirrhosis) or post-hepatic (e.g. tumour compression). As there is a rich collateral supply to the abdominal viscera, a substantial rise in portal pressure will cause the formation of porto-systemic anastomoses. The most clinically significant of these are oesophageal varices, which can present with life-threatening gastrointestinal bleeding. Splenomegaly can occur secondary to backpressure through the splenic vein and may cause leukopaenia, thrombocytopaenia and anaemia.

Diaphragmatic varices can complicate surgery at the time of liver transplantation and may cause subphrenic haematomas that may become secondarily infected and form abscesses.

43 a. The arterial blood gas (ABG) results provided in this question are all within the normal range. The patient has an adequate PO2 without retaining carbon dioxide. These results suggest that 35% of oxygen is adequate for this patient; lower levels may not provide adequate oxygenation and higher levels may lead to CO2 retention. A baseline ABG will have already been performed on air and therefore this is not necessary to repeat. It is important to repeat a blood gas sample on 28% oxygen as this may also provide suitable results. Having established the most appropriate oxygen

180

concentrations it is sometimes useful to measure saturations after exercise to ensure that no drop is seen in the level of oxygenation. This patient went on to have lung function tests, which in addition to a PaO2 $\updownarrow$ 7.3kPa on air meant that he satisfied the criteria for long-term oxygen therapy.

44 e. Examination skills can be learned by rote to a large extent although an experienced candidate will be slick in their approach. Interpretation of clinical findings proves to be more of a challenge for students. In this case we are provided with three pieces of clinical information:

$\downarrow$ chest expansion unilaterally.

$\downarrow$ breath sounds on the affected side.

$\downarrow$ percussion note on the affected side.

These features are all leaning towards a diagnosis of an extensive collapse or pneumonectomy. A lobectomy would be unlikely to provide such dramatic signs as the remainder of the lung normally expands to fill the void left by removal of a single lobe.

Characteristic findings of a pleural effusion would be $\downarrow$ chest expansion on the affected side, stony dullness to percussion with bronchial breathing above the effusion. Other scenarios are widely available in clinical textbooks although there is no substitute for clinical practice for compounding your knowledge!

45 a. Flow volume loops can be difficult to interpret for the inexperienced student. The x-axis represents time, whilst the y-axis is a measure of both inspiratory and expiratory flow (the negative deflection is the inspiratory component whilst the positive is expiratory measured in litres per second.). Flow volume loop **a** shows a typical loop of a person that does not suffer with respiratory disease. The expiratory curve shows maximal peak expiratory flow and the straight line joining up to the inspiratory curve suggests a non-collapsible airway. Curve **b** represents a patient suffering with emphysema. The expiratory curve shows early airway collapse, the inspiratory phase is reduced in volume compared with our normal patient. Curve **c** represents fixed upper airways obstruction whilst **d** represents variable upper airways obstruction and curve **e** shows a restrictive pattern.

46 d. *Streptococcus pneumoniae* is the commonest cause of community-acquired pneumonia. Students are often under the misconception that the organism most likely to be responsible for community-acquired pneumonia is *Staphylococcus aureus*. This is responsible for most hospital-acquired pneumonias. *Haemophilus influenzae* is the second most common organism responsible for community-acquired pneumonia.

181

Patients suffering from chronic obstructive pulmonary disease are most likely to get chest infections caused by Moraxella catarallis due to their underlying lung condition.

47 c. Antibiotic use in community-acquired pneumonia varies with GP preference. The recommended antibiotic for a simple case is amoxicillin (provided that the patient is not allergic to penicillins). Amoxicillin is derived from ampicillin which is better absorbed, producing higher plasma and tissue concentrations, and whose absorption is not affected by the presence of food in the gut. Augmentin is a compound preparation of amoxicillin and the beta-lactamase inhibitor clavulanic acid. The clavulanic acid protects the amoxicillin from the penicillinases produced by virtually all staphylococci and therefore this should not be given as first-line therapy since *Staphylococcus* is not one of the most common infective organisms. Metronidazole provides cover for anaerobes and works by breaking DNA strands. Erythromycin may be used in patients with allergies to penicillins.

48 a. While several other species of genus *Legionella* have been identified, *L. pneumophila* is the most frequent cause of human legionellosis and a relatively common cause of community-acquired and nosocomial pneumonia in adults. The organism can be found in natural aquatic habitats (freshwater streams and lakes, etc.) and artificial sources (cooling towers, potable water distribution systems). *Legionella* organisms are cleared from the upper respiratory tract by mucociliary action. Any process that compromises mucociliary clearance (e.g. smoking) increases risk of infection. *Legionella* organisms may infect other parts of the body including the lymph nodes, brain, kidney, liver, spleen, bone marrow and myocardium.

Staphylococcus aureus is usually a hospital-acquired pneumonia and pneumococcal pneumonia will usually present as a lobar infiltration.

49 b. There are two significant congenital diaphragmatic abnormalities that usually require intervention: (1) large central tendon defects and (2) herniation through the foramen of Bochdalek. Congenital herniation of abdominal contents through the foramen of Morgagni are usually small and insignificant and usually require no further treatment. Trauma to the diaphragm can occur with both blunt or penetrating injury to the abdomen and usually affect the relatively unprotected left hemidiaphragm.

The liver usually takes the brunt of right-sided injury resulting in relative right hemidiaphragm sparing. These usually require urgent surgical intervention as fulminant respiratory distress is likely to occur. Embryologically the diaphragm is made up of the septum transversum, pleuroperitoneal membrane, mesentery of the dorsal oesophagus and the dorsal body wall, neatly summed up by the mnemonic 'Several

182

Parts Make Diaphragm'.

50 a. Being of female sex affords a certain amount of resistance to the development of duodenal ulceration and this is markedlyseen during pregnancy. Steroid use has been shown to predispose to the formation of ulcers by mechanisms that involve both a disturbance in acid regulation and secretion and interference with the normal protective mucosal layer of the stomach.

Cushing's ulcer is the eponymous name given to the devel-opment of acute peptic ulceration secondary to head injury, major surgery or acutely stressful conditions, and a strong association between ulcer formation and severe burns has also been described (Curling's ulcer). These findings form the basis for the routine use of proton pump inhibitors such as omeprazole as part of the gastrointestinal prophylaxis of the critical care bundle in situations of acute stress.

51 e. Post-operative ileus is a common recognised sequel of abdominal surgery where handling of the bowel leads to a period of inactivity. It is commonly seen in open as opposed to laparoscopic procedures due to the greater manipulation of the bowel required in this type of approach. The initiation of oral intake is often subjective and will depend on factors such as the length of operation, the difficulty of the procedure, i.e. a case of ruptured appendix will normally accompany a greater period of bowel inactivity than an intact but inflamed appendix. Anastomotic leak is a serious complication more often seen during large bowel procedures due to the relatively poor blood supply to this part of the gastrointestinal tract. It is usually heralded by a tense, rigid abdomen, absence of bowel sounds and a patient who is unwell. Adverse reactions to anaesthetic agents are relatively common, however, usually present soon postoperatively or soon after induction of anaesthesia. Small bowel obstruction can be a long-term complication of any abdominal surgery, however, is almost never the cause of such a clinical picture so soon after appendicectomy.

52 d. The prescription of anti-emetic medication should always be with caution; the cause for vomiting should be assessed and a diagnosis made before starting anti-emetics. Serious causes for vomiting, e.g. gastrointestinal obstruction, must be excluded.

Erect chest radiographs are useful if perforation is suspected; however, in this case the clinical index of suspicion is low and would not be a useful investigation. Abdominal radiographs are useful only in cases of suspected gastrointestinal obstruction, as a crude assessment of renal tract stones (a KUB – kidneys, ureter, bladder radiograph is far superior) and often as a useful method of confirming constipation in elderly patients whocomplain of abdominal pain and difficulty in passing stool!

Nasogastric tube passage would be an option if vomiting were severe or unlikely to settle with anti-emetics. However, it would not be necessary to feed a patient like this via nasogastric tube in the short term and thus would be an unnecessary hindrance to recovery of normal oral intake. Proton pump inhibitors such as omeprazole are not required in a young patient without documented peptic ulcer disease and in this example would not afford any significant benefit in the immediate management of vomiting caused by post-operative ileus.

53 a. The diagnosis is strongly suggested by two salient features in the history: the presence of high blood glucose in an elderly man with no previous history of diabetes mellitus and jaundice. Compression of the distal end of the common bile duct by the head of the pancreas causes backpressure leading to jaundice. The presence of new-onset diabetes mellitus in the elderly should always be treated with suspicion and a diagnosis of diabetes mellitus should never be made until an attempt to rule out malignancy has been undertaken. Cholangiocarcinoma does present with weight loss, jaundice and deranged liver enzymes; however, the presence of raised blood glucose with a painless hepatomegaly is more suggestive of head of pancreas cancer. Choledocholithiasis (literally stone in biliary tree) can cause an intermittent jaundice and right upper quadrant pain, however weight loss and hepatomegaly suggest a more sinister cause. Hepatitis is usually associated with tender hepatomegaly and does not usually accompany raised blood glucose.

54 b. Chest radiography is the investigation most likely to aid with diagnosis of the cause of breathlessness. The history is consistent with an element of heart failure with peripheral as well as pulmonary oedema; however, a large unilateral pleural effusion should raise suspicion of a localised respiratory lesion, e.g. infection or malignancy. An echocardiogram will not be useful diagnostically as the clinical signs point to a degree of heart failure and an electrocardiogram, although a useful screening tool for suspected pulmonary embolus and signs of cardiac disease, can be performed later once localised disease has been ruled out.

Pleural tap and drainage are the most useful diagnostically and therapeutically, however, in the non-acute situation radiographic confirmation of the diagnosis and extent of pleural effusion is useful. Finally, there is a tendency to start antibiotics empirically in elderly patients without accurate history of diagnosis. The minimal history and examination are not strongly suggestive of pneumonia and it is sensible to await chest imaging before considering antibiotics.

55 e. Scaphoid fracture. This injury is one of the most commonly injured bones of the carpal row, thought to be due to the higher stresses imposed on the scaphoid due to its unique position spanning both proximal and distal rows of the carpal bones. Falling on an outstretched hand is the mechanism of injury usually encountered in this type of injury, occasionally complicated by neurovascular compromise as with any fracture. Tenderness in the anatomical snuffbox forms a useful clinical reckoner if scaphoid fracture is suspected.

56 a. This history is representative of Crohn's disease. It is a chronic inflammatory condition of the GI tract, it is characterised by transmural granulomatous inflammation. Crohn's disease may affect any part of the gut from the mouth to the anus, but favours the terminal ileum and proximal colon. Unlike ulcerative colitis there are parts of the bowel that are unaffected in between lesions. Ulcerative colitis does not have skip lesions; 15% of patients have a positive family history and there is an increased risk in smokers of 3–4 times. Extra-intestinal signs include erythema nodosum, clubbing, conjunctivitis, episcle-ritis and arthritis among others. Investigations include blood tests, sigmoidoscopy and biopsies and small bowel enema.

Exacerbations are managed with intravenous steroids and rehydration with topical treatment if necessary.

57 e. This lady is suffering with toxic shock syndrome. It was first described in 1978 and is caused by the exotoxin *Staphylococcus aureus*. In extreme cases the condition may progress onto *Streptococcus* multi-organ failure. Other clinical symptoms include a fluctuation in the level of consciousness and a widespread erythematous macular rash. The biggest clue to the diagnosis comes from the history of recent menstruation and useful investigations include vaginal examination, blood tests for U&Es, LFTs, clotting screen, FBC and arterial blood gas. Other useful tests include an ECG and a chest X-ray to exclude other causes of these symptoms.

58 d. *Gardnerella vaginalis* produces an offensive brown discharge, it causes an inflammation of the vagina in women or the glans penis in men. It often results in dysuria. Both chlamydia and gonorrhoea result in urethritis. Whilst most infections can be distinguished by colour or quality of discharge the most reliable method is by taking appropriate swabs.

59 d. The prevalence of disease is defined as the number of active cases in a defined time divided by the total population surveyed.

The number of people with the disease is 20,000 people in that year with the total population in the same period being 140,000. Incidence is defined as the number of new cases diagnosed in given time period divided by the total population in that time period. Thus option **b** (500/140,000) describes the incidence of the disease.

Option **e** (250/140,000) describes the mortality rate specific to that disease. A similarly calculated figure is the absolute mortality rate (sometimes referred to as the death rate), which describes the total number of deaths per population.

60 e. An upper motor neurone paralysis is usually seen as a result of a stroke. It results in weakness of the facial muscles but spares the muscles of the forehead due to their dual innervation. The facial nerve arises from its origin in the pons and travels past the cerebello-pontine angle through the petrous part of the temporal bone to emerge via the stylomastoid foramen into the parotid gland where it divides into branches. Along its course it traverses with the chorda tympani and the nerve to stapedius, therefore if there is a lesion in the petrous temporal bone the facial weakness is accompanied by hyperacusis and loss of taste on the affected side.

Bell's Palsy is by far the commonest cause of a lower motor neurone lesion and is a diagnosis of exclusion. It is believed to result from a viral infection and results in swelling of the nerve in the petrous temporal bone. The absence of symptoms in any of the other cranial nerves helps to secure the diagnosis.

Management involves time and most patients make a full and spontaneous recover over a period of months.

Extended matching questions

61 d. This scenario is describing a dislocation of the hip. This is commonly caused by trauma to the leg including a dash board injury during a road traffic accident or injury involving a motorbike. From the examination the important features to remember are the positioning of the leg, although shortening is seen in both fractures and dislocations, internal rotation is characteristic of posterior dislocations of the hip. In cases of fractures or dislocations patients may well experience difficulty in weight bearing after the injury and therefore this does not distinguish one from the other. The other possible diagnosis in this case is a peri-prosthetic fracture, this will usually be clearly visible on X-ray if it is present.

62 a. This child is suffering with an irritable hip. Many hip conditions in children have similar presentation during their early stages and thus are difficult to distinguish. The commonest cause responsible for this condition is a transient synovitis which usually resolves within a couple of weeks. In a child of this age it is important to consider other paediatric conditions including Perthes' disease and slipped upper femoral epiphyses although both of these would have some positive findings on X-ray. Although his hip joint does not feel hot nor does it look erythematous the possibility of a septic arthritis needs to be investigated. This is done by a battery of blood tests including inflammatory markers and aspiration of the joint. In children, and particularly in the case of a hip joint this aspiration is best done under general anaesthetic in the operating theatre.

The fluid obtained should be urgently sent to microbiology for microscopy, Gram staining and culture.

63 b. This patient has suffered a fractured neck of femur. This diagnosis should always be considered in elderly patients with a history of falls, particularly in those patients who are unable to weight bear due to pain. There are different types of neck of femur fractures and their management varies in accordance with the type of fracture sustained.

Fractures may be either intracapsular or extracapsular.

Intracapsular fractures

These are is divided by the level of the fracture line in the neck:

• Subcapital

• Transcervical

• Basal

In this group, the proximal fragment often loses part of its blood supply and hence the union of this fracture is difficult. This is a serious injury in the elderly patient. In the very old and debilitated person, it can precipitate a crisis in the precarious metabolic balance. It can become a terminal illness due to uraemia, pneumonia, bed sores, etc., and be fatal.

Extracapsular fractures

These are all grouped as trochanteric fractures of various types.

Patients with intracapsular fractures are managed by hemiar throplasty whilst extracapsular fractures are managed with a dynamic hip screw.

64 e. This lady has suffered a peri-prosthetic fracture. In patients undergoing any kind of procedure involving insertion of prostheses this is a potential risk. It is believed that some of these fractures are caused at the time of insertion although, they are too small to be picked up at the time, it is only when they become symptomatic they are discovered. It is a particular complication with the resurfacing prosthesis – should this happen the management involves removing the prosthesis and inserting a more traditional hip replacement. For patients complaining of such symptoms so soon after surgery peri-prosthetic fractures should be considered as a potential differential diagnosis.

65 h. In this scenario the diagnosis is of a septic arthritis until proven otherwise. He has a fever and severely limited range of movement in the affected joint which are characteristic findings of a septic joint. It is normally said that the joint should be hot and swollen though in the case of the hip it is not possible to assess these findings due to the depth of the joint itself.

The raised white cell count and inflammatory markers confirm the diagnosis and the ultimate way to do this is by aspirating a sample from the joint. In the case of the hip this is often done under general anaesthesia. In this particular case, if the metalwork has become infected it is more than likely that it will need to be removed and occasionally replaced.

66 a. Cocaine is a pre-synaptic reuptake inhibitor effectively increasing the synaptic concentrations of dopamine, noradrenaline and serotonin at higher doses. Dopamine is involved in the so-called 'reward' pathways of the brain and hence higher levels lead to the feeling of euphoria and 'high' that is produced by cocaine use. Cocaine is also a vasoconstricting drug and this action can be seen with disastrous effect in those individuals who swallow packets of cocaine with subsequent eruption of the packets in the gastrointestinal tract. Massive local vasoconstriction can occur leading to ischaemic segments of bowel as well as systemic absorption leading to tachycardia (due to increased sympathetic drive), myocardial ischaemia due to vasoconstriction and tachycardia (termed rate-related ischaemia) that may manifest as angina and increased risk of stroke due to hypertension and localised ischaemia due to vasoconstriction followed by reperfusion injury.

The local anaesthetic effect of cocaine (it was for many years used as a topical anaesthetic agent) when applied systemically can cause conduction defects in the myocardium and arrhythmias and these must be borne in mind when treating patients with suspected cocaine overdose. Aspirin must not be used in the acute management of angina-like pain as the risk of cerebral haemorrhage post-vasoconstriction is high and bleeding can be catastrophic.

67 i. Marijuana (*Cannabis*) is the most commonly abused illicit substance in the United States. It has a variety of actions that vary from euphoria, an altered perception of space and time, hallucinations, anxiety and paranoia to drowsiness and with chronic use the development of an 'amotivational syndrome' characterised by a lack of interest in social and occupational life and a lack of energy. The mechanism of effect of marijuana is still largely unknown although the putative active agent is delta-L-tetrahydrocannabinol (THC), correlating to large numbers of diverse THC receptors found scattered throughout the brain. Long-term effects include orthostatic hypotension and tachycardia and smoking marijuana has been linked with the development of a lung disease similar to chronic obstructive pulmonary disease. Effects on the central nervous system are controversial but appear to include a type of atrophy that may be related to long-term use. Frequently seen are the injected conjunctiva of marijuana use.

68 g. Chronic alcohol use has been linked to various vitamin and essential mineral deficiencies due to both a lack of dietary intake and secondary to vomiting. Most notable are the effects of a lack of thiamine and vitamin B12, which are involved in the development of Wernicke's encephalopathy and Korsakoff's psychosis and when chronic can lead to subacute degeneration of the spinal cord (vitamin B12). This lady is exhibiting signs and symptoms of Wernicke's encephalopathy – a triad of ataxia, ophthalmoplegia and confusion, and may progress to the irreversible Korsakoff's psychosis manifests as confabulation and memory deficits. The ECG changes are most likely due to hypomagnesaemia, occasionally seen in alcoholics, those with malabsorption syndromes and diabetics. The widened QT interval has been linked to a risk of developing torsade de pointes and correction of the electrolyte deficit should be part of the standard of care for the acute management of complications of chronic alcohol abuse.

69 f. Opioids are responsible for a plethora of adverse effects if   abused the most serious of which is respiratory depression. This can often be so severe as to cause a life-threatening depression that may occur whilst the patient retains a level of consciousness. Miosis, nausea, vomiting, constipation, itch and hypotension are some of the other effects that are suggestive of opioid overdose. Florid respiratory depression may manifest clinically as a very low respiratory rate causing a drop in pH as CO_2 is not cleared and a loss of consciousness (hence the high CO_2 and low pH suggesting a respiratory acidosis in this scenario).

Easily reversed by opioid antagonists such as naloxone and naltrexone the clinician must not be lulled into a false sense of security by the apparent improvement in the patient's clinical state as the effects of some of the longer-lasting opioids (such as methadone) and large doses can quickly overcome the effects of such antagonists.

70 d. PCP is a powerful dissociative hallucinogen originally used as an anaesthetic agent until the post-anaesthesia side-effects associated with the drug

189

precluded its use. When abused it has been associated with psychosis, violence and agitation,

tachycardia and high temperature and anxiety. Neurological signs such as vertical or horizontal nystagmus are common as is hypertension. Tachypnoea and irregular breathing patterns have been described in PCP users and rarely muscular rigidity syndromes and dystonias are seen. Treatment modalities aim to reduce absorption via the gastrointestinal tract when ingested and to reduce the agitating effects of the drug. Benzodiazepines are a safe antidote to control the behavioural symptoms associated with use and are preferable to antipsychotic agents, which carry the risk of causing neuroleptic malignant syndrome, seizures and malignant hyperthermia. Rhabdomyolysis is a side-effect of muscular rigidity syndromes and merits testing of creatinine kinase levels and careful monitoring of renal function with aggressive fluid therapy if suspected.

71 f. Bacterial vaginosis, although a cause of vaginal discharge, is not usually classified as a sexually transmitted infection as it can present unrelated to sexual intercourse. The terminology vaginosis is used as there is usually no inflammation of the vagina, separating this condition from diseases causing vaginitis. A change in the normal pH of the vagina is thought to play a role in the alteration of the normal flora and encourages overgrowth of bacteria such as *Gardnerella vaginalis*, *Mycoplasma hominis*, *Mobiluncus* spp. and anaerobes such as *Bacteroides*.

Microscopy of vaginal epithelial cells reveals the presence of 'clue cells', which are squamous vaginal cells on which the causative bacteria are attached.

72 g. Gonorrhoea typically presents in men with a yellow purulent discharge from the urethra with associated dysuria and irritation.

However, *Neisseria gonorrhoea* has a predilection for epithelium of the cervix, rectum, conjunctiva and pharynx depending upon exposure to such sites. In women the presentation is much more subtle and insidious. Up to 50% of women may be asymptomatic with gonorrhoea and may eventually present with altered vaginal discharge, dysuria and intermenstrual bleeding with fertility problems as a long-term consequence of severe untreated infection. *Neisseria gonorrhoea* exists as Gram-negative intracellular diplococci and are easily recognisable on microscopy. Treatment involves using fluoroquinolones such as ciprofloxacin or ofloxacin for uncomplicated disease, amoxicillin (sometimes with probenecid) in penicillin-sensitive areas or ceftriaxone in areas of high penicillin resistance.

73 a. *Candida albicans* is an extremely common non-sexually transmitted infection of females and males. In females it can cause a very itchy vulvovaginal rash (pruritus vulvae) with a creamy white curd-like discharge from the vagina. In men infection with *Candida albicans* may occasionally arise due to cross-infection from a partner but more usually is the manifestation of an underlying disorder such as immunosuppression, diabetes or over use of broad-spectrum antibiotics. In this case the patient was a known diabetic and some would argue that the routine work-up of male patients presenting with balanitis (infection of thehead of the penis) should include investigation of undiagnosed diabetes. Treatment can be obtained over the counter as either a topical antifungal pessary or cream or as an oral tablet.

74 c. *Chlamydia trachomatis* is a common sexually transmitted infection with up to 5% of the UK population of sexually active women infected. It is often clinically silent until the long-term consequences are discovered and a retrospective diagnosis is offered. Some authorities report figures as high as 80% for asymptomatic infection in women with approximately half of all infected males demonstrating no clinical symptoms. Well recognised sequelae of infection with *Chlamydia trachomatis* are infertility (due to salpingitis and pelvic inflammatory disease) and Reiter's syndrome – a triad of conjunctivitis, arthritis and urethritis. Diagnosis of *Chlamydia trachomatis* is complicated by the fact that it is an obligate intracellular bacterium and thus complex cell culture, direct fluorescent antibody and DNA testing form the mainstay of diagnostic techniques.

75 b. TV is a sexually transmitted infection that causes inflammation of the vagina (vaginitis) and can often be confused with bacterial vaginosis (BV) a non-sexually transmitted infection that does not affect the vagina itself. The discharge is classically described as a 'champagne discharge' as it is green-yellow and frothy and may accompany a 'strawberry cervix' – so-called as the cervix is often dotted with small haemorrhagic areas. Diagnosis is with dark-ground microscopy on a wet prepar-ation and treatment involves metronidazole 400mg twice daily for a week.

76 a. Reiter's syndrome presents classically with a triad of urethritis, conjunctivitis and arthritis. It is sometimes sub-classified as part of reactive arthritis, which presents similarly after a gastrointestinal infection. Reiter's syndrome typically affects young males with a sexually transmitted infection such as non-specific urethritis. Joint involvement is limited usually to a few large joints.

77 g. Psoriatic arthropathy may present with a range of arthritis patterns, the most common of which is arthritis affecting the distal interphalangeal joints. Evidence of nail changes is very strongly suggestive and manifest as nail pitting, nail dystrophy and onycholysis (lifting of the nail from the nail bed). For reasons still not entirely clear, between 5% and 8% of individuals with psoriasis develop a seronegative arthritis. Radiologically, the erosions of psoriatic arthropathy are central in the joint and present

191

with thinning of the distal end of a phalanx (pencil) in a relatively spared proximal end of the adjacent phalanx (cup) giving a pencil-in-cup appearance.

78 h. Enthesopathy is an inflammation at the junction of ligament or tendon and bone and it occurs more frequently with seronegative arthritides than other arthritides, e.g. rheumatoid arthritis. Typically presenting as plantar fasciitis or Achilles tendonitis patients usually complain of pain and stiffness at the affected site. The pathogenetic basis of enthesopathy is still not known; however, molecular mimicry and cross-reaction between infective organisms and joint components are thought to play a role.

79 d. Ankylosing Spondylitis (AS) is more common in males than females and presents with back pain, morning stiffness, decreased thoracic excursion, chest pain as well as extra-articular features such as uveitis, enthesopathy and rarely aortitis.

A reduction in back flexion to less than 5 cm as assessed by Schoeber's test in a young male with sacroiliac pain is almost diagnostic of ankylosing spondylitis. Radiological changes are marked with local erosion of bone at the junction of spinal ligament and bone with bone healing at these sights (syndesmophyte formation) causing ankylosis (fusion) of the vertebrae.

AS and other spondyloarthritides are all associated with the HLA-B27 subtype.

80 b. Enteropathic arthropathy can be seen in between 10% and 15% of sufferers of ulcerative colitis and Crohn's disease.

As with many of the seronegative arthritides the joints are affected in an asymmetrical pattern with the large lower limb joints preferentially affected. Interestingly the arthritis symptoms may occur some time before the gastrointestinal disturbance. Gastrointestinal bypass surgery has also been linked to the development of an arthritis picture similar to that associated with inflammatory bowel disease and is thought to be due to the introduction of antigens normally protected from the immune system by changes in the normal mucosal uptake of the gastrointestinal tract as a consequence of surgery.

81 f. Although there are several conditions that could mimic this history the most serious is a Wilm's tumour. They arise from the kidneys and may present with haematuria. Due to the nature of their presentation, these tumours can often become large before producing any symptoms or signs. Any patient with a suspected malignancy or suggestion of a mass should be sent for appropriate imaging, either CT scanning or ultrasound with an appropriate surgical referral made in anticipation of the result.

82 a. This vignette is describing a case of intussusception. Itaffects children between the ages of 6 months and 4 years old and results in abdominal pain. Since the affected children are young they often appear to be unwell, occasionally vomit and characteristically pass red currant jelly-like stool. Other clinical features include a fever and a palpable abdominal mass.

Abdominal X-rays may appear to be entirely normal or may show an absent caecal shadow. Diagnosis may be confirmed or indeed managed by air or barium enema, it characteristically reveals a coiled spring or sudden termination of barium. These patients should be urgently referred to the surgical team.

83 d. The case in question is describing volvulus. This occurs when a segment of bowel rotates on its mesentery resulting in obstruction and abdominal distension with associated pain. There is an association with congenital malrotations but it can occur in other scenarios including adhesions from previous surgery or Meckel's diverticulum. The best management involves a high index of suspicion with rapid abdominal X-ray and surgical referral in order to preserve viable bowel.

84 b. This is a case of pyloric stenosis. It is most common in first born males and most frequently occurs between the ages of 2 and 10 weeks. Vomiting is characteristically projectile in nature with progressive dehydration and constipation. The vomiting is unaltered food and in severe cases a hypochloraemic acidosis may be seen. On examination a palpable mass in the epigastrium may represent the thickening of the pylorus – it is most easily felt during a feed. The diagnosis can be confirmed on ultrasound scan and surgical management is necessary to relieve the obstruction.

85 e. Acute appendicitis should always be considered in a child presenting with acute abdominal pain with fever. Although in this case it is important to be cautious that her symptoms do not relate to her reproductive tract. Further probing in the history revealed commencement of the pain in the centre of the abdomen some 24 hours earlier with radiation of the pain down

to the right iliac fossa. Gynaecological causes of pain tend to originate in the appropriate iliac fossa. To confirm the diagnosis an ultrasound scan should be obtained as this can be useful in excluding diagnoses such as ovarian cysts in addition to confirming appendicitis.

86 a. The mechanism of action of atropine is via blockage of the vagus nerve and subsequently enhances sinus node automaticity and atrioventricular conduction:

193

• Atropine causes blockade of parasympathetic activity at both the sinoatrial (SA) node and the atrioventricular (AV) node it may increase sinus automaticity and facilitate AV node conduction.

• Dosages of atropine for adults in asystole, or pulseless electrical activity with a rate less than 60 beats per minute, is 3 mg i.v..

Atropine may increase myocardial oxygen demand and unmasksympathetic overactivity.

87 e. The dose of magnesium sulphate is 8 mmol (4 mL of a 50% solution) for refractory ventricular fibrillation if there is any suspicion of hypomagnesaemia, especially if the patient is on potassium-losing diuretics.

Other indications are for the use of magnesium are:

• Ventricular tachyarrhythmias in the presence of possible hypomagnesaemia.

• Torsade de pointes.

Digoxin toxicity.

88 c. The use of amiodarone in shock-refractory VF is believed to improve survival. Experts believe that in VF or pulseless VT resistant to three shocks there is a role for amiodarone. Initially 300 mg intravenously should be given before continuing with shocks. The UK Resuscitation Council suggests that a further dose of 150 mg may be given for recurrent or refractory VF/VT followed by an infusion of 900 mg over the next 24 hours.

89 f. Adenosine slows conduction across the atrioventricular (AV) node but has limited effect on myocardial cells, this makes it very effective for terminating paroxysmal supraventricular tachycardias associated with re-entrant circuits. Adenosine has a short duration of action and therefore the affect of the drug may be short-lived. Induction of AV nodal block can reveal underlying atrial rhythms in those patients presenting with narrow complex tachycardias, it slows down the ventricular response. Side-effects of administration of adenosine include episodes of severe bradycardia.

90 h. Flecainide is a potent blocker of sodium channels and therefore slows conduction. The effect of flecainide can be seen on the ECG as lengthening of the PR interval and widening of the QRS complex.

Flecainide is known to be negatively inotropic and may result in bradycardia and

194

hypotension. Other side-effects documented include blurring of vision and oral paraesthesiae.

PAPER 3 ANSWERS

Answers and notes

Multiple choice questions (single best answer)

1 a. Alport's syndrome is an inherited disease of the kidney affecting young boys between 5 and 20 years of age. Inheritance is in three forms: X-linked dominant, autosomal dominant or autosomal recessive. The clinical presentation is one of asymptomatic haematuria with progressive sensorineural deafness and eye disorders (lenticonus). Treatment is to support the progressive renal failure. Renal transplantation may be considered, however, there is a risk of anti-glomerular basement membrane nephritis even after transplantation. Anderson–Fabry disease is anX-linked-recessive disorder of trihexoside deposition. Clinical features include a burning sensation in distal limbs associated with a characteristic blue hued rash (angiokeratoma corporis diffu-sum). Goodpasture's syndrome is a pulmonary–renal syndrome manifest as pulmonary haemorrhage and massive haemoptysis associated with proliferative glomerulonephritis. Linear anti-glomerular basement membrane deposits are seen on immunofluorescent staining of biopsy specimens. Treatment involves aggressive immunosuppression with or without plasmapheresis.

Wegener's granulomatosis is a necrotising granulomatous vasculitis affecting the respiratory tract and kidney. Typically sinusitis with epistaxis, haemoptysis and renal failure all co-exist.

Autoantibody assay returns a positive anti-neutrophil cytoplasmic antibody (c-ANCA), which responds to corticosteroid and cyclosphosphamide. Von Hippel–Lindau syndrome is an oncologic vascular disorder manifest in many different organs with renal cysts and tumours, phaeochromocytoma, retinal angiomas and haemangioblastomas of brain and spinal cord being most frequently seen. Clinical clues to the diagnosis are often posterior fossa symptoms of dizziness, ataxia and headache in young adults often with retinal detachment detectable on fundoscopy.

2 d. Myeloma should always be kept in mind when considering the differential diagnosis of an elderly patient with back pain and renal failure. The simple and non-invasive urine test for Bence–Jones protein, the light-chain fragment of the B-cells overexpressed in myeloma, makes this investigation one that should not be overlooked in the diagnostic work-up of patients with renal failure. The mechanism of renal failure in myeloma is thought to be a directly toxic effect of light chains on the nephrons and

196

leads to the characteristic 'flea-bitten' appearance of myeloma kidney.

Paget's disease is a disorder primarily of bone remodelling leading to alternating osteoclastic bone resorption followed by abnormal osteoblastic woven bone formation. Symptoms usually include bone pain, excessive warmth over the affected bony sites due to hypervascularity, bony deformity and neuropathy due to nerve compression (especially the vestibulocochlear nerve). Sarcoidosis is characterised by the presence of non-caseating granulomata and is most classically a disease of the respiratory system, however, renal involvement is seen in rare cases. Hyperparathyroidism can lead to a raised calcium and is usually seen as the byproduct of failing kidneys. However, chronic hyperparathyroidism itself may manifest as renal stones, uraemia and eventual renal failure. Bony involvement is common and may be seen as an erosive arthropathy, subperiosteal bone resorption at the phalangeal tufts or a 'rickets-type' picture. Osteosarcoma presents typically with pain and soft tissue swelling and classically Codman's triangle is seen on radiographs, indicative of periosteal tenting from underlying bone. Radiographic appearances are usually a mixed lytic sclerotic picture but purely lytic or sclerotic lesions can be seen.

3 c. Caeruloplasmin and serum copper are useful tests in the investigation of liver disease of unknown aetiology and are sensitive indicators of the presence of Wilson's disease (hepatolenticular degeneration). A renal ultrasound scan is useful to identify any obstruction, scarring from previous infection or altered renal size indicative of long-term renal damage or chronically reduced renal blood flow. Safe and non-invasive to perform this should always be considered in the investigation of renal disease. Complement levels (C3 and C4) as well as double-stranded DNA (dsDNA) and erythrocyte sedimentation rate (ESR) should be used as a screen for systemic lupus erythematosus (SLE, lupus) nephritis. Generally, an elevated ESR and anti-dsDNA and low C3 and C4 levels are associated with active nephritis. Anti-neutrophil cytoplasmic antibodies (ANCA) are useful in the detection of vasculitic diseases affecting the kidney such as Wegener's granulomatosis and Churg–Strauss disease among many. Bence–Jones protein (light-chain fragment) is a simple and effective screening tool for suspected myeloma with associated light-chain nephropathy and should never be omitted from the diagnostic work-up of renal failure.

4 a. Renal ultrasonography should be the first-line investigation of those listed. Other useful investigations to be considered initially should be a urine dipstick, urine pregnancy test and a bedside blood glucose level. Blood pressure is markedly elevated in this otherwise well middle-aged woman and the deterioration in renal function is significant. The additional clue from the history that two relatives suffered strokes at a 'young age' should prompt strong consideration of a diagnosis ofautosomal-dominant polycystic kidney disease (ADPKD). ADPKD is associated with cerebral (berry) aneurysms, cysts in other organs such as liver, pancreas and spleen and cardiac valvular defects.

Renal failure is progressive and may lead to end-stage renal disease (ESRD). Renal ultrasound scan is a very sensitive and specific tool in detecting cystic abnormalities of the kidneys and may well confirm the suspected diagnosis. CT scan of the head should not be rushed into on the basis of a lack of neurological signs until other simple investigations have been performed and would only be indicated if blood pressure control did not ameliorate symptoms. Renal biopsy is not without serious risks and should never be undertaken unless knowing histology will influence management; 24-hour urine collection for metanephrines is indicated in cases of suspected phaeochromocytoma and along with adrenal CT scanning aids diagnosis of this rare cause of hypertensive crisis. Carotid and vertebral Dopplers are sometimes indicated in cases of stroke secondary to suspected arterial stenosis such as atherosclerotic disease. A history of multiple transient ischaemic attacks (TIA) or strokes in the absence of a good cause such as atrial fibrillation may prompt examination of carotid arterial flow waveform. A similar process may occur in the vertebrobasilar system (so-called posterior circulation stroke) and manifests as symptoms of dizziness, vertigo, nausea and lower cranial nerve abnormalities.

5 c. This question has slightly different answers depending on practice in North America or other parts of the world, however, the main message is the same. Surgical exploration of both kidneys with histopathological diagnosis is the gold standard for focussing future treatment. In Europe imaging modalities may suffice for a firm diagnosis of unilateral versus bilateral disease to be made with an operative approach favoured in borderline cases. In North America there is a trend towards early operative diagnosis with exploration of both kidneys. CT scanning of the abdomen has a role in the diagnosis of a suspected Wilm's tumour, however, staging CT of the chest, abdomen and pelvis must be performed to assess for metastatic spread of tumour. Renal ultrasonography may initially be used to assess for tumour involvement, however, it does not carry the sensitivity nor specificity of CT or MR imaging. Chest radiography is a useful baseline investigation to assess for pulmonary metastases but again if Wilm's tumour is identified then staging CT is performed. Albumin/creatinine ratio is a very useful investigation in the work-up of renal disease of various origins and can detect microalbuminuria (defined as the presence of albumin in the urine of 30–300 mg/day) – one of the pathological hallmarks of early renal disease. Especially useful in the investigation of patients with diabetes and cardiovascular disease it should be performed on a regular basis to guide secondary prevention strategies, e.g. tight blood pressure or glucose control and as a prognostic indicator of the level of renal deterioration.

6 c. Drug-induced interstitial nephritis presents acutely typically following commencement of penicillins although it has been described in association with diuretics such as frusemide, non-steroidal anti-inflammatory drugs (NSAIDS) and sometimes with infections. Acute renal failure associated with fever, arthralgia, rash and eosinophils in both blood and urine help to make the diagnosis. Haemolytic uraemic syndrome (HUS) is a vascular disorder with the formation of platelet aggregates. A triad of symptoms are usually seen (i) microangiopathic haemolytic anaemia (ii) thrombocytopaenia and (iii) acute renal failure. It is the commonest cause of acute renal failure in children and usually occurs following a diarrhoeal disorder although many infections may cause HUS. Cholesterol embolus is rarely seen but can be catastrophic when occurring. Clinically manifest with disturbance of renal biochemistry associated with eosinophilia and purpura of limbs usually in those with arterial disease. A net-like rash (livedo reticularis) is sometimes described similar to that seen in systemic lupus erythematosus (SLE) and may aid diagnosis.

Acute tubular necrosis is a common and spontaneously resolving cause of acute renal failure and is associated with hypovolaemia, drugs that are nephrotoxic and rhabdomyolysis by a direct insult to the renal tubules from excess myoglobin in the glomerular filtrate. The typical clinical picture is of acute renal failure refractory to rehydration that eventually responds within days to weeks. Treatment is to ensure adequate hydration until tubule function is restored.

7 e. Head injuries may result in basal fractures to the petrous temporal bone which can result in damage to the seventh cranial nerve. Although uncommon cranial sarcoid may be bilateral and can affect cranial nerves III, V, VI and VII. Lyme disease is caused by infection via tics and the infective organism is Borrelia Bergdorfori. The commonest neuropathy associated with this condition is of the facial nerve and can once again be bilateral.

Gullain–Barre syndrome is usually symmetrical and ascending in its presentation. In severe cases cranial nerves may be involved although in less severe cases its pathology remains in the limbs and trunk. Medullary infarction results in damage to the nucleus of cranial nerve VII which provides upper motor neurone signs.

8 d. Holmes–Adie pupil is usually large but can be small after prolonged light exposure. In acute retrobulbar neuritis pupils are of normal size, often an afferent defect may be seen on the affected eye. Amitriptyline overdose gives large pupils due to the anti-cholinergic effect. Unequal pupils or anisocoria is seen in syphilis. Pontine haemorrhage gives a bilateral sympathetic lesion probably associated with parasympathetic overactivity resulting in constricted pupils.

9 b. A spastic paraparesis is usually seen in upper motor neurone lesions. It is a fairly common feature of multiple sclerosis often due to plaques affecting the cervical and thoracic cord. In the case of syringomyelia, the syrinx acts as a mass effect often affecting the cervical cord resulting in upper motor neurone signs most commonly in the legs with a wasting and weakness affecting the trunk and arms in a cape-like distribution. In the case of a meningioma the symptoms are caused by a mass effect.

Since the spinal cord terminates at the level of L1-2 any pathology affecting the lumbosacral spine will result in lower motor neurone signs and therefore weakness would be seen most commonly.

10 e. Hypercalcaemia may result in vague limb pains but not muscle cramps. A low calcium may account for twitching or tetany as will hyponatraemia or hypokalaemia. Cramps have been reported in cases of hyponatraemia. Central pontine myelinolysis usually results from a rapid correction of hyponatraemia, the neurological symptoms that develop are believed to be secondary to oedema of the cells in the pons. Hyperthyroidism is known to result in proximal limb myopathies, tremor, hyper-reflexia and occasionally seizures as can hyponatraemia. A rare complication of hypoglycaemia is hemiparesis. It is occasionally seen in infants and children but is easily treatable with intravenous glucose which normally results in a complete recovery.

11 c. The nerve supply to the thenar muscles of the hand is the median nerve whilst, the nerve supply to the intrinsic small muscles of the hand is supplied by the ulnar nerve. A lesion of the ulnar nerve at the elbow would result in damage to the hypothenar and small muscles of the hand but would have no effect on the thenar eminence. Syringomyelia provides weakness and muscle wasting in a cape-like distribution and wasting in the arms is a fairly common peripheral symptom of ALS.

Whilst osteoarthritis of the lower cervical and upper thoracic spine is uncommon, it does occur and would result in similar problems to those defined in this case.

12 a. Creutzfeld–Jakob disease is caused by a mutation in a naturally occurring in a prion protein. A typical presentation is by a progressive dementia and psychiatric symptoms. The new form of the disease is thought to be much slower in its onset developing over the course of a few years rather than a few months. Although a link to infected meat is a suspected cause this has not been confirmed but there is evidence to suggest that infection may be transmitted by surgical procedures and corneal transplants. Whilst imaging may provide diagnostic information tonsillar biopsy provides a tissue diagnosis.

13 a. CEA may be raised in gastrointestinal cancers, especially colorectal carcinoma. As with all tumour markers it can be raised in a variety of cases, notably pancreatitis, cirrhosis and smoking, and must be interpreted within the clinical context. Tumour markers should never be used as a diagnostic tool; the use of markers is to add weight to an already strong clinical index of suspicion and to help guide investigation of possible sites of neoplasm. CA19-9 is also associated with colorectal cancer, however, it may also be raised in pancreatic cancer. AFP is most specific for hepatocellular carcinoma but also may rise in germ cell tumours as well as other liver disorders. NSE is specific for small cell carcinoma of the lung and HCG is raised in pregnancy (depending on your point of view possibly the most benign cause of a distended abdomen) as well as germ cell tumours. CA 153 is raised most commonly in breast disorders including cancer and benign breast disease.

14 b. HIDA scan is a nuclear medicine scan involving intravenous injection of a 99mtechnetium-labelled derivative of iminodiacetic acid. It is an invaluable scan in the investigation of bile duct leakage post-operatively. The radionuclide is excreted by the liver into the biliary system and through into the duodenum. Imaging is taken serially after injection and will define the gallbladder to duodenum in hours. Identification of leaks is evident as nuclear uptake in areas external to the biliary system. HIDA scan has an additional purpose in the identification of acute cholecystitis and has a sensitivity of around 96% and a specificity of around 94%. The easily performed and non-invasive ultrasound examination of the gallbladder has, however, rendered HIDA obsolete as a first-line investigation for the diagnosis of cholecystitis. Plain abdominal radiograph will not detect a bile leak, however, it may be useful in showing air in the biliary tree as may occur with conditions such as choledo-chal fistula seen in gallstone ileus and with gas-forming organism infection of the biliary tree. CT scan of the abdomen will detect hepatic abnormalities such as cysts, tumours and collections but is poor at visualising the biliary system and will not demonstrate bile leak. ERCP is both a diagnostic and therapeutic tool for imaging the biliary and pancreatic tree, however, is not as sensitive as HIDA as demonstrating bile leak.

15 d. This clinical picture points towards a lung abscess. Most frequently, the lung abscess arises as a complication of aspiration pneumonia caused by mouth anaerobes. Abscesses can be primary or secondary in origin. A primary abscess is infectious in origin, caused by aspiration or pneumonia in the healthy host whilst a secondary abscess is caused by an underlying condition (e.g. obstruction), spread from an distal site, bronchiectasis and/or an immunocompromised state. It is possible to classify ascesses by the infectious organism, e.g. *Staphylococcus* lung abscess and anaerobic or *Aspergillus* lung abscess.

In this clinical scenario the important factors to identify are the swinging fever and the recurrence of cough with foul smelling sputum shortly after a chest infection. These are both factors that should raise suspicion of an abscess. In addition, the X-ray findings of a walled cavity should raise the possibility of the diagnosis. Empyema is different as it is inflammatory fluid and debris within the pleural space. It may result from an untreated pleural space infection which subsequently progresses collection in the pleural space.

16 b. Bronchiectasis is the abnormal and permanent distortion of one or more of the conducting bronchi or airways, most often secondary to an infectious process. It can be catagorized as a chronic obstructive pulmonary lung disease manifested by airways that are inflamed and easily collapsible, which in turn results in air flow obstruction and impaired clearance of secretions. It may be congenital or acquired, although the congenital form is normally diagnosed during childhood. The condition results in destruction of muscular and elastic component of the bronchial walls, which impairs mucociliary clearance and predisposes to recurrent infections.

Impaired clearance of secretions causes colonisation and infection with pathogenic organisms, contributing to the common purulent expectoration noted in patients with bronchiectasis. The result is further bronchial damage and a vicious cycle of bronchial damage, bronchial dilatation, impaired clearance of secretions, recurrent infection and more bronchial damage.

Diagnosis is usually based on a compatible clinical history of chronic respiratory symptoms, such as a daily cough and viscid sputum production, as well as typical findings on CT scan.

17 d. There are many causes of round opacities on chest X-rays.

Their location may provide a clue to the likely diagnosis but often it is necessary to revert back to the history and examination for clues. Tuberculosis tends to present in the apices due to the apparent improved oxygenation. Both lung cancer and carcinoid tumour can present anywhere in the lung fields as round lesions.

Sarcoid is a multi-system disorder characterised by non caseating epithelioid granulomas. Other commonly involved organ systems include the lymph nodes; the skin; the eyes; the liver; the heart; and the nervous, musculoskeletal, renal and endocrine systems. Patients usually complain of non-specific symptoms including weight loss and fatigue. Chest symptoms are fairly common amongst sufferers of the disease.

18 e. Syndrome of inappropriate anti-diuretic hormone secretion is associated with small cell lung cancer. Release of anti-diuretic hormone results in the dilution of the serum, which in turn gives a relative hyponatraemia. Depending on the location of the lung cancer, local spread can include applying pressure onto the superior vena cava resulting in reduced blood return to the heart from the upper half of the body. The superior vena cava is the major drainage vessel for venous blood from the head, neck, upper extremities and upper thorax. It is located in the middle mediastinum and is surrounded by relatively rigid structures such as the sternum, trachea, right bronchus, aorta, pulmonary artery, and the perihilar and paratracheal lymph nodes. It is a thin-walled, low-pressure, vascular structure. This wall is easily compressed as it traverses the right side of the mediastinum.

Clinical features include venous distension of the neck and chest wall, facial oedema, upper extremity oedema, mental changes, lassitude, cyanosis and even coma.

Pressure on the recurrent laryngeal nerve can result in a palsy of the vocal cords and a hoarse voice whilst growth into the sympathetic system can lead to a Horner's syndrome, ptosis, meiosis and anhydrosis on the ipsilateral side.

Pulmonary oedema is not a complication of lung cancer.

19 e. Respiratory failure is a syndrome in which the respiratory system fails in one or both of its gas exchange functions: oxygenation and carbon dioxide elimination. Respiratory failure may be classified as hypoxaemic or hypercapnic and may be either acute or chronic.

Hypoxaemic respiratory failure (type I) is characterised by a low PaO_2 with a normal or low $PaCO_2$. This is the most common form of respiratory failure, and it can be associated with virtually all acute diseases of the lung, which generally involve fluid filling or collapse of alveolar units. Some examples of type I respiratory failure are cardiogenic or non-cardiogenic pulmonary oedema, pneumonia, acute pulmonary embolus and acute exacerbation of asthma.

Hypercapnic respiratory failure (type II) is characterised by a low PaO_2 and a high $PaCO_2$. The pH depends on the level of bicarbonate, which, in turn, is dependent on the duration of hypercapnia. Common causes include drug overdose, neuromuscular disease, chest wall abnormalities and severe airway disorders (e.g. asthma, chronic obstructive pulmonary disease (COPD) and chronic pulmonary emboli).

20 c. Major risk factors for pulmonary emboli include:

• Immobility.

• Abdominal/pelvic surgery.

• Malignancy (abdominal/pelvic/advanced metastatic).

203

• Lower limb fracture.

• Pregnancy.

• Hip/knee replacement.

• Previous venous thromboembolism.

Minor risk factors include:

• Oral contraceptive pills.

• HRT.

• Long-distance travel.

21 d. Liver failure presents with a plethora of physical signs: jaundice, fluid shift leading to pulmonary oedema and effusion, ascites and peripheral oedema and biochemical derangement of liver function, e.g. increased clotting time, decreased protein/immunoglobulin synthesis, etc. Fluid collections associated with liver failure tend to be transudates rather than exudates (transudates ↕30g/dL protein; exudates □30g/dL).

'**Ex**udates **Ex**ceed 30 g/dL protein' is one way of remembering the association. Transudates are mainly associated with *failures*: **1.** Heart failure.

2. Liver failure.

3. Kidney failure (nephrotic syndrome).

4. Thyroid failures.

On the contrary, exudates are mainly associated with:

1. *Infection* (e.g. pneumonia, TB).

2. *Inflammation* (e.g. rheumatoid arthritis, SLE).

3. *Malignancy* (e.g. bronchial carcinoma, lymphoma and mesothelioma).

The most likely diagnosis from the pleural tap would be

malignancy in this case and must be excluded.

22 d. Midline shift is a warning sign of raised intracranial pressure and eventual herniation of brainstem through the foramen magnum. Colloquially known as cerebral compartment syndrome any space-occupying lesion such as tumour, infection, bleeding, etc. may cause a rise in the pressure inside the closed space with catastrophic effect. Modalities used for treating non-surgically amenable causes of raised intracranial pressure include: (1) raising the head of the bed to 30 degrees, (2) osmotic diuresis with mannitol, (3) thiopentone infusion and (4) hyperventilation (rarely performed). Extradural haematoma evacuation is a priority in cases of proven midline shift and/or localising signs (e.g. pupillary inequality).

Neuroradiological clipping or coiling of intracerebral aneurysm is not indicated here as the source of bleeding is external to the brain itself.

23 a. Respiratory distress is a complication of upper torso burns that must be closely monitored. Surgical escharotomy may be required to release the mechanical restriction to breathing caused by circumferential burns to the chest wall. Infection may result in the intervening period as wound breakdown occurs but does not present such an emergency. Loss of peripheral pulses is again treated with surgical release of constricting tissues most often associated with circumferential burns of the limbs and may influence the decision to transfer an otherwise stable patient to a specialist burns unit rather than at a general treatment centre. Acute stress ulceration (Curling's ulcer) is managed with proton pump inhibition and has been robustly shown to be effective in treating this complication. Severe dehydration is a close second for the most important complication to be vigi-lant for in severe burns, however, younger patients can tolerate a larger degree of fluid loss than the elderly. A rough indication to prognosis following burns can be estimated by using the formula below:

patient's age

⬚ % burn ☐ 100 ⬚ poor chance of survival e.g. 48-year old ⬚ 35% burn ⬚ 83 i.e. moderate chance of survival

24 b. The growth of male breast tissue, known as gynaecomastia, is a normal finding in the neonate due to maternal oestrogens, and the pubertal boy and elderly male due to the changing ratio of testosterone to oestrogens in these age groups. This is not a typical finding that would be consistent with non-accidental injury and therefore a referral to social services would be inappropriate.

Referral to a breast surgeon and needle aspiration are also unjustified in this case and may even be deleterious to growing breast tissue. Short-course prednisolone is also unwarranted and is not indicated in cases of gynaecomastia.

25 e. Ureteric obstruction is confirmed clinically by an intravenous urogram (IVU). In up to 90% of cases the causative stone can be seen on X-ray of the kidneys, ureter and bladder (KUB) and this is recommended prior to undertaking an IVU as contrast may obliterate from view a small but otherwise radio-opaque stone. Delayed excretion and dilatation of ureter or renal

pelvis are useful in making the diagnosis and are frequently seen in this investigation. Reduction in kidney size is not due to obstruction of the outflow tract with the opposite often the case. Perfusion defects can occur in cases of inflow limitation such as renal artery stenosis but will not occur due to outflow obstruction. Bladder residual volumes are rarely seen in cases where a stone has travelled the length of the urinary tract and lodges distal to the neck of the bladder.

26 c. Adhesions post-surgery and strangulated hernias are the most common causes of obstruction of the bowel and therefore are not to be missed when assessing a patient. Classically small-strangulated femoral hernias are missed in obese elderly women.

Ulcerative colitis is a disease affecting the colon with the exception of backwash ileitis and would not considered as a cause of small bowel obstruction in this woman. Gastro-colic fistulae can occur in Crohn's disease but more commonly lead to faeculent vomiting than obstruction. Intussusception is a disease affecting typically 5–12-month-old infants. Meckel's diverticulum can lead to small bowel obstruction but this is rare and the most common presentation is one of inflammation.

27 a. He is suffering from rheumatic fever. This infection remains common in the Third World although it is a dreaded complication of a streptococcal sore throat in the West. Diagnosis is made on a group of criteria.

• *Major criteria*:

– Carditis – tachycardia or new murmurs.

– Arthritis – usually a migratory arthritis.

– Subcutaneous nodules.

– Erythema marginatum – rash with raised red edges and a clear centre.

– Sydenham's chorea.

• *Minor criteria*:

– Fever.

– Raised ESR or CRP.

– Arthralgia.

– Prolonged P-R interval.

– Previous rheumatic fever.

Using the revised Jones' criteria there must be evidence of a recent *Streptococcus* infection and 2 major criteria **or** 1 major and 2 minor criteria.

28 b. This vignette represents a clinical picture of coarctation of the aorta. In this picture there is narrowing of the aortic lumen just distal to the subclavian artery. This results in left ventricular hypertrophy as a result of increased afterload and hypertension secondary to reduced renal perfusion. The reduced blood flow results in the mottled appearances of the lower limbs.

Cyanosis does not usually occur in this condition unless the patient is severely anaemic.

29 c. This girl is suffering from pelvic inflammatory disease. This disease ascends from the cervix to the uterus and the fallopian tubes. On examination it is common to find a low-grade pyrexia with lower central abdominal pain. There may be associated nausea and vomiting with tenderness on vaginal examination with cervical excitation commonly exhibited; 90% of there infections are sexually transmitted and the commonest age group to be involved is those between 15 and 20 years of age. The commonest causative organism is *Chlamydia trachomatis* but *Neisseria gonorrhoea* is often implicated. Following pelvic inflammatory disease there is a 5 times increased risk of developing an ectopic pregnancy and infertility.

30 a. 90% of cervical cancers are squamous. Of the remaining 10% the majority are adenocarcinoma. It is a disease that is heavily screened for but symptoms are all too often ignored by those affected. There is a national screening programme in which all women aged 25 years and over (or younger in socially deprived areas) are invited to attend a 3 yearly screening program. There is currently a vaccine under trial for Human

Papilloma Virus (HPV) although, it is in the clinical trial stage at present. A common presentation is intermenstrual bleeding or post-coital bleeding which should always prompt an internal examination and speculum. Any patient that has an abnormal looking cervix should be referred to the local gynaecological service for further review and testing.

31 e. The Chi-squared test is most often used in situations where raw data is being examined for effect and is similar to the paired t-test in generating p values, however, the latter is used for comparison of the means of two populations. p value generation describes the number generated by calculation of the squared difference between the observed and expected values as a fraction of the expected values. This value is then converted to a p value relative to the degrees of freedom associated with the number of rows and columns involved.

p values are useful determinates of whether an observation (or set of observations) generated is likely to be due to chance. For example, setting a p value of less than 0.05 is often taken to herald significance (meaning that you are confident that there is only a 5% risk that the data is due to chance events rather than the ordered effect of a true measurable difference). Limits for significance cutoff can be set at higher or lower levels such that in a small population it may only be appropriate to use a cut-off value of less than 0.01, i.e. 1% to attain significance, although this may be in practice difficult to achieve.

Positive predictive values refer to the predictive power of a test and is defined as the number of true positives who tested positive for a disease. It is a useful method of assessing the accuracy of a test and as it is linked to the prevalence of a disease in a population (number of active cases per population per unit time) it will become more reliable with higher prevalences (due to reduction of the statistical error generated by small sample size).

Odds ratio is used to approximate the relative risk of an event occurring and is used most often in examining data from case-control studies.

The Mann–Whitney

U-test is a non-parametric test that compares two unpaired groups, that is to say that they do not have to follow a normal distribution and the variance within the population from which the data are selected does not have to be equal.

The test compares two medians to assess whether the samples are from the same population or not. For simplicities sake it is essentially a non-parametric, i.e. does not have the same con-straints on population variance and distribution as the t-test but

208

allows a comparison to be made between two data sets.

32 c. Although radiologically the cervical spine X-rays are clear and clinically the patient complains of no tenderness it is important that a CT scan of her neck is organised urgently and her neck is kept immobilised in the meantime. The key feature in this history is the fractured distal radius and iliac wing as well as the history of a fall from a height of approximately 15–20 feet.

Having sustained other serious injuries this patient is not in a position to confirm or deny any cervical spine tenderness. In the presence of distracting injuries further imaging should be sought before removal of cervical spine protection. If you ever have any doubts the case should always be discussed with a senior colleague as the consequences of any error is potentially life threatening.

33 d. Loss of pulse is a very late sign of compartment syndrome.

If not suspected before this sign is present, the outcome is likely to be poor. Signs of compartment syndrome include:

1. pain in the affected limb disproportionate to the injury, **2.** pain on passive movements of the affected limb,

3. pallor,

4. paralysis (often difficult to asses due to presence of cast), **5.** paraesthesiae.

If there is any doubt about the integrity of a compartment the intra-compartmental pressure should be measured. As a guide, if it is greater than 40 mmHg urgent treatment, e.g. fasci-otomy, should be considered. If you suspect a diagnosis of compartment syndrome senior review should be sought.

34 d. Patients have the right to be fully informed about their diagnosis in order that they may make informed decisions about their medical care. In the case of patients who are assessed to be competent this should always be the principle upon which to act.

In very special situations where the release of a diagnosis is very strongly thought to be seriously detrimental to the health of the patient (and advice from psychiatrists and ethics departments and close communication with the family is strongly advised) then a diagnosis may be withheld from a patient although these cases are few and far between and should only be made by the consultant in charge of that patient's care.

It is required of a doctor who has requested an investigation under implied, verbal or written consent (such as laboratory tests or a chest radiograph, etc.) to disclose the results of that investigation as and when the results become available in a timely manner such that the patient is given adequate time and information to make an informed choice regarding their care. For example, informing a patient that they are to receive a blood transfusion for anaemia on the basis of blood results known the day before surgery 10 minutes from the time of surgery is not appropriate.

Leaving decisions to break bad news to other health care providers who were not responsible for ordering the diagnostic investigation is also not appropriate (e.g. requesting an HIV test on a medical inpatient and asking the GP to break the news of a new diagnosis of HIV).

Additionally, although family members may be involved

closely in the care of their relatives with the consent of the patient, it should not be left to the family to disclose results of investigations or aspects of medical care with the patient without a doctor discussing these directly with the patient. The responsibility of a doctor caring for a patient does not extend to the family and the relationship should be confidential and exclusive unless explicitly expressed by the patient themselves.

As a useful rule of thumb in the clinical setting, if there is ever any doubt regarding the appropriateness of an interaction then the patient's right to absolute confidentiality to the treating team(s) directly involved in their care must be preserved and consent to extend that confidentiality to include other members must be authorised by the patient themself.

35 e. Dapsone is a sulpha-derivative drug that is employed in the effective treatment of dermatitis herpetiformis. Treatment modalities used in the management of psoriasis include agents to keep the skin hydrated such as moisturisers and emollients, cold tar, topical steroids and vitamin D analogues and vitamin A analogues such as tazarotene. Erythrodermic or acute generalised pustular psoriasis is one of the few true dermatological emergencies and should be initially managed with topical treatments and immunosuppressants such as methotrexate and cyclosporin.

Cold tar has anti-inflammatory properties that make this most effective in treating chronic plaque psoriasis, however, patient concordance with treatment is poor. Systemic treatments are also employed to managed chronic stable psoriasis and guttate psoriasis and may consist of ultraviolet light therapy or photo-chemotherapy such as PUVA (**p**soralen plus **u**ltra**v**iolet **A** light), which can be effective in almost all kinds of psoriasis.

36 a. The presentation is strongly suspicious for scabies and in this age group should be high on the differential of an itchy rash.

Scabies is caused by the *Sarcoptes scabiei* mite, which has a predilection for the epidermis. Typical features of scabies are of an intensely itchy rash, which is caused by a delayed type hypersensitivity reaction to the mite itself, with characteristic inflammatory papules and almost pathognomonic burrows or tracts.

Areas commonly affected include the hands and feet with fin-

gers, wrists and webspaces, the most often afflicted. Treatment modalities include one or two applications of malathion or permethrin cream, which are left on the skin for a period of 12 or 24 hours. Aqueous cream is used in the treatment of eczema and whilst it may give some mild symptomatic relief, is not effective in treating scabies. Flucloxacillin 500mg 3 times daily is usually given in conjunction with another penicillin derivative for cellu-litic infections. If a viral infection was suspected in a young child it may be appropriate to adopt a conservative management policy, however, this will not lead to adequate symptom control and resolution in scabies. Cold tar is a very effective but messy treatment option in the management of psoriasis and acts as an anti-inflammatory agent when applied topically to psoriatic areas.

37 b. The history above is describing a case of pyelonephritis. The features of the vignette suggesting more than a simple urinary tract infection include the systemic signs of fever, tachypnoea, low saturations and tachycardia. In this case the blood results also showed a raised white cell count with a creatinine of 468

suggesting an acute renal failure secondary to the pyelonephritis. This lady made a good recovery with a combination of i.v. fluids and reduced doses of gentamycin and timentin. Since she experiences systemic symptoms oral antibiotics with community follow-up would be an inadequate management plan, although catheterisation and analgesia are important adjuncts to her therapy, alone they are insufficient.

38 d. In patients with bowel cancer urinary symptoms are fairly common. The mass effect from the bowel mass exerts pressure on the urinary system which causes urinary retention. This may subsequently result in a urinary tract infection due to stagnation of urine but the initial symptom is one of difficulty in instigating urination. In those patients undergoing either elective or emergency bowel surgery it is of vital importance that a catheter is inserted to keep the bladder decompressed at all times and to prevent any stagnation in the system. Bowel cancer doesnot metastasise to the prostate gland and bladder cancer usually results in painless haematuria as a presenting symptom as opposed to dysuria.

39 d. The protein content of the fluid aspirated from the pleural effusion is consistent with a transudate. Causes of transudates can be grouped together as 'failures' e.g. cardiac failure, liver failure (cirrhosis), renal failure (nephrotic syndrome) and thyroid failure (hypothyroidism). Exudates are defined by a protein content greater than 30g/L and caused by infections (e.g. pneumonia), inflammations or malignancies (e.g. bronchial carcinoma).

40 c. Vomiting in meningitis is due to raised intracranial pressure and is central or neurogenic in origin. Patients may offer this clue to the cause of their vomiting by stating that the episode of vomiting came as a surprise to them and was not preceded by a period of nausea. Other causes of neurogenic vomiting are centrally acting drugs and any other cause of raised intracranial pressure such as space-occupying lesion. The other options, whilst feasible, are less likely to be the cause of vomiting in an otherwise healthy young man. NSAID-associated gastritis would be more likely to occur in an elderly patient but more often presents insidiously as an iron-deficient anaemia or occasionally as melaena.

41 d. The case describes a history of a transient ischaemic attack, there is no residual neurological deficit 24 hours after onset of symptoms. Risk factors for TIAs include: male sex, age, smoking, diabetes, hypercholesterolaemia, hypertension and past history of cardiovascular disease. This gentleman had his carotid vessels scanned which showed an 80% stenosis which means that he is at a high risk of developing a further TIA or CVA in the following months. With these findings on carotid scanning the patient should be referred to a vascular surgeon with a view of doing a carotid endarterectomy to reduce the chances of an embolus being dislodged.

42 a. Haloperidol is an extremely useful medication for the acute management of a confused patient with agitation and behavioural symptoms. An alternative agent used to manage behavioural effects of dementia is risperidone, which shares a similar incidence of Parkinsonism side-effects but is more expensive than haloperidol. Given orally, intramuscularly or intravenously these are effective first-line medications for the treatment of acute behavioural crises.

Benzodiazepines should be avoided in demented patients due to the paradoxical exacerbation of behaviour and sedation that occurs. In the acute setting a demented patient should never be assumed to suffer from intrinsic dementia until all organic and reversible causes have been ruled out. A nice mnemonic for tying in the causes of dementia is 'DEMENTIAS' – standing for **D**egenerative diseases (Parkinson's disease, Huntingdon's disease, Alzheimer's disease), **E**ndocrine disorders, **M**etabolic derangement, **E**xogenous factors (heavy metals, drugs, medications), **N**eoplasia, **T**rauma (e.g. subdural haematoma), **I**nfection, **A**ffective disorders (e.g. pseudo-

212

dementia) and vaScular (vascular dementia, ischaemic stroke and vasculitis).

Memantine is an NMDA antagonist used in the treatment of cognitive symptoms of Alzheimer's disease. It may be most effective when used in conjunction with cholinesterase inhibitors such as galantamine and rivastigmine. These medications act to increase acetylcholine levels, thought to be the biological correlate responsible for memory and concentration. There is evidence that the cholinesterase inhibitors may ameliorate the so-called secondary (behavioural) component to Alzheimer's disease, however, they are not appropriate for use acutely in the demented patient.

Olanzipine and the other atypical antipsychotic agents are effective agents when used as maintenance of behavioural disturbance, however, are not as predictable in effect when used acutely and thus tend to accede to the 'older' neuroleptic medications such as haloperidol and risperidone.

Sertraline is a selective-serotonin reuptake inhibitor (SSRI) and is a useful adjunct in the treatment of depressive symptoms associated with dementia. It has a good side-effect to treatment profile and may have some benefit for psychotic disturbance as well as mood disturbance.

43 b. The tricyclic antidepressants have a recognisable pattern of toxicity that occurs in overdose, which can be summed up as the 'Tri-C's of toxicity' – **C**onvulsions, **C**oma, **C**ardiac arrhythmias. Patients may present asymptomatically having been found by someone close to the patient or they may sometime self-refer to hospital feeling remorseful of their actions, however, seriousside-effects may be delayed for between 2 and 6 hours post-ingestion and careful monitoring should be undertaken of anyone suspected of having an overdose. Cardiac monitoring is essential due to the inhibition of normal cardiac conduction (due to inhibition of the fast sodium channel) leading especially to a prolonged QT interval. Anti-cholinergic effects are also seen commonly with overdose of the tricyclics due to their potent competitive antagonism at central and peripheral muscarinic acetylcholine receptors.

Monoamine oxidase inhibitors (MAOI) such as tranylcypromine when taken in overdose usually manifest with symptoms of catecholamine excess (e.g. sweating, tachycardia, hypertension, tremours and seizures) but arrhythmias are typically uncommon in the setting of pure MAOI ingestion.

A well-recognised phenomenon occurring in individuals who are prescribed MAOIs is a hyperadrenergic state resulting from the ingestion of foods containing tyramine such as cheese, red wine and some meats and is due to the build-up of tyramine in the presence of MAOIs (as it is not broken down due to the enzyme inhibition) and acts as a sympathomimetic.

213

A similar phenomenon known as a serotonin syndrome may occur in individuals co-prescribed MAOIs and selective serotonin reuptake inhibitors (SSRIs) or even those who overdose with SSRIs (e.g. sertraline) with symptoms of flushing, a change in mental status, sweating and hyperthermia as well as neuromuscular agitation may occur.

Beta-blockade usually causes symptoms of bradycardia and hypotension, which may be life threatening. Other effects less commonly seen are bronchospasm in sensitive individuals and hypoglycaemia in diabetics. The agent of choice to reverse beta-blocker overdose is glucagon, which seems to act independently of the beta receptor to increase heart rate and myocardial contractility.

Digoxin toxicity is manifest by a yellow-green colour disturbance to normal vision, confusion and/or agitation in addition to the distinctive 'reverse tick sign' on electrocardiography. Premature ventricular contractions (PVCs), bigeminy and trigeminy are often encountered signs of digoxin toxicity.

Hypokalaemia, hypomagnesaemia and hypernatraemia can all potentiate digoxin toxicity even at normal therapeutic doses and should be considered as a cause of toxicity. Reversal is by use of digibind (a digoxin-binding antibody).

44 a. The diagnosis in this case is of Hodgkin's disease. Approximately 80% of patients with this condition test positive for Epstein–Barr virus. The condition occurs in young fit people and the elderly. There is an increased risk in those family members of the affected patient. Symptoms are divided into categories A and B where B include constitutional symptoms such as weight loss and night sweats. The diagnosis is confirmed by lymph node biopsy. Treatment depends on the staging and location of the lymphoma.

45 a. The mean age of presentation of myeloma is 65–70 years of age. Myeloma has a clone of cancerous plasma cells which fill the bone marrow and produce a paraprotein M. The production of normal immunoglobulin is suppressed which results in an increased risk of developing infection. Anaemia is a common finding due to chronic disease as is renal failure. Bone marrow normally produces equal amounts of light and heavy chains which make up the immunoglobulin ratio, in myeloma more light chains are produced (Bence–Jones proteins). The median survival is approximately 3 years and disease control is achieved in over half of patients with melphalan. Allogenic bone marrow transplant has been used in small number of young patients with a 25% success rate. Myeloma has a characteristic blood picture including:

↑ **Calcium**

Normal phosphate

Normal alkaline phosphatase

46 b. This question is difficult only because it requires a knowledge of the genetic translocation associated with the more familiar *bcr–abl* fusion gene (Philadelphia chromosome). Genetic translocations are responsible for a large number of genetic predispositions to cancer. Another commonly seen translocation associated with cancer is the t(8;14) *c-myc* activation leading to an increased risk of developing Burkitt's lymphoma. A handy way to remember the chromosomes involved in the Philadelphia chromosome is as follows. Philadelphia chromosome – the 'P' of philadelphia is located at the 9th position and there are 22 letters in the two words put together (hence 9;22). The t(11;22) translocation is commonly associated with a rare bone tumour seen almost exclusively in children and young adults. It is a highly malignant tumour that has a high mortality rate in those who are afflicted.

Robertsonian translocations are a type of genetic transfer of chromosomal material that occurs in association with a number of disorders, most commonly with Down syndrome.

Robertsonian translocations can be balanced, in which case there is no loss or addition of chromosomal material and the person carrying that karyotype will be a carrier of Down syndrome and not be afflicted, or unbalanced, resulting in trisomy or monosomy (the latter of which is non-viable). Down syndrome involves trisomy of chromosome 21 and may involve a combination of nearby chromosomes. The translocation t(14;21) is relatively frequently identified as the cause of this disease.

47 c. This question is included to remind the clinician that the management of disease should always remain with the patient as a central focus. The indicators specified may all be associated with disease activity, although the role of early involvement of biological agents is currently being evaluated. Subjectively from a patient's perspective the useful function that is managed comfortably in rheumatoid arthritis is the best indicator of disease activity. Appearances are often deceiving with 'normal' radiographs disguising disabling pain and loss of function whilst long-term deformities of the hands may mask surprising dexterity and adaptation.

48 d. Antiphospholipid syndrome is a spectrum of systemic lupus erythematosus (SLE) often associated with vascular thromboses. The vascular involvement may manifest most strikingly as stroke, myocardial infarction and multi-infarct dementia in a younger population with no obvious identifiable risk factors or more insidiously with migrainous symptoms and recurrent miscarriages. The presence of lupus anticoagulant and anticardiolipin antibodies with the above clinical presentation strongly suggests antiphospholipid syndrome. Reiter's syndrome typically presents with a triad of

215

urethritis, conjunctivitis and arthritis in a young man associated with sexually transmitted or gastrointestinal infections. Systemic sclerosis is a disorder mainly affecting skin, gastrointestinal tract and respiratory system whilst dermatomyositis, as the name suggests, affects skin and muscle mainly. Marfan's syndrome typically affects the aorta and aortic valve, lens of the eye and skeletal system due to mutations in the fibrillin-1 gene.

49 a. The most likely diagnosis in this case is a fibroadenoma of the breast. It is most commonly seen in women age between 15 and 40 years old. Characteristically, fibroadenomas are smooth, firm and well-circumscribed lumps. They may vary in size from 1 to 5cm and are often very mobile. Along with all other breast lumps these should be investigated using the triple approach and their management, if small, should include reassurance. For larger fibroadenomas management may include excision to restore symmetry to the breasts. Approximately 30% of fibroadenomas shrink and disappear completely. There is no association between fibroadenomas and breast cancer.

50 b. The most likely cause for this gentleman's gynaecomastia is liver failure. The history states that he has suffered with pancreatitis and acute liver failure in the past which suggest that this is likely to be due to hepato-biliary failure. Although it is a physiological change seen in the elderly, this gentleman's condition is most likely to be secondary to further liver problems.

There is no evidence that he is suffering with thyroid dysfunction and the history does not state that he is on any medications that are known to cause this condition including digoxin, steroids, methyldopa and anti-androgens.

51 b. Acute glaucoma is a common condition affecting the elderly and one of the few true ocular emergencies that presents acutely. Classified as acute angle-closure and open-angle glaucoma, pain is typically unilateral and may be associated with headache. Blurred vision and visual distortion are symptoms experienced frequently and may be severe enough to reduce acuity to recognition of hand movements only. Dim light,anti-cholinergic drugs and intrinsic anatomical predisposition such as a shallow anterior chamber all predispose to acute angle-closure glaucoma and may be relieved by drugs reducing aqueous humour production such as beta-blockers and acetazolamide.

A few doses of a topical steroid preparation may aid in dampening the inflammatory response that accompanies glaucoma.

Endophthalmitis describes an intra-ocular inflammation usually caused by infection affecting the aqueous or vitreous humour and may occur as a result of direct

216

inoculation of infectious agent to the eye (e.g. foreign body penetration) or endogenously via spread from a pre-existing primary focus. Systemic antibiotics are usually indicated for infectious causes and may be treated adjuvantly by administration of antibiotic and steroid directly into the eye. Involvement of an ophthalmologist is always indicated and should be performed immediately once the diagnosis is suspected. Retinitis pigmentosa is a complex inherited disorder of the retinal photoreceptors and pigment epithelium. There is a slight male predominance in afflic- tion due to the more frequent X-linked varieties. Loss of night vision and peripheral vision are the most common complaints in those affected. Treatment modalities have been shown to

have modest benefit and are mainly involved in symptom control. These include massive vitamin A dosing, the use of acetazolamide along with experimental procedures such as retinal prosthesis or transplantation. Retinal detachment may occur as a result of traction from retinal neovascularisation with attachment to the vitreous humour, a tear in the surface with mechanical detachment by subretinal vitreous humour invasion or as a result of vascular changes in the retina (e.g. hypertension or vasculitis). The sensation of flashing lights and floaters associated with patches of lost vision (scotomata) are the most commonly described phenomenon. Retinal artery

occlusion usually presents with painless sudden loss of vision in one eye and is caused by emboli. The pathophysiology is similar to that of cerebral stroke. There may be a role for thrombolysis if an embolus is detected within the first 4–6 hours but the mainstay of treatment is expectant management with investigation of the underlying cause.

52 e. Hyperglycaemia and diabetes has been linked to the development of posterior subcapsular cataract by a mechanism thought to be due to chronic osmotic changes, modification of lens protein and oxidative damage in the lens. A distortion in vision can often be experienced with accumulation of high blood glucose levels and is often complained of in patients who present with hyperosmolar hyperglycaemic and diabetic ketoacidotic states and who experience large and often rapid shifts in the osmotic content of the lens whilst on treatment.

Steroids, hypertriglyceridaemia, obesity and hypertension have all been demonstrated to be associated with this type of senile cataract at a young age. Posterior subcapsular cataracts tend to present with more florid and disabling visual disturbance than cortical, nuclear or mixed cataracts (the other subclas-sifications of senile cataracts). Glare, especially in sunlight or with bright headlights at night, reduction in visual acuity and sometimes a reduction in accommodation. Treatment is primarily surgical with lens extraction and replacement providing great improvement in vision. Cataract operations have become almost standard procedures in day surgery units and can be performed with complete removal of the lens (intra capsular cataract extraction, ICCE) or with removal of the lens nucleus only with retention of the posterior capsule (extracapsular cataract extraction, ECCE). ECCE is the currently preferred method of extraction, however, the choice of procedure depends on the surgeon, patient and the type of cataract present.

53 d. Amiodarone is a drug notorious for its detrimental effect on the lungs, thyroid and liver and is best remembered for these derangements by the mnemonic 'PFTs, LFTs and TFTs.'

Amiodarone can cause a picture of hyperthyroidism as it is structurally similar to thyroxine and thus thyroid function tests must be monitored on a regular basis with a low threshold to stop or reduce dosing if thyroid derangement is detected. Pulmonary fibrosis and skin manifestations such as photosensitivity reactions have also been reported. Atorvastatin has been linked to myositis (like all the statin drugs) and attention to the development of muscle pain and weakness should prompt assessment of dosing and or consideration of changing to another statin or other class of lipid-regulating drug. Statins must be used with caution in hypothyroidism due to the increased risk of myositis with untreated hypothyroidism and correction of thyroid dysfunction may itself lead to an amelioration of lipid profile. Amlodipine is associated with many diffuse symptoms including gastrointestinal upset but the main problem with use is the development of ankle swelling, which may only partially respond to diuresis.

Atenolol and other beta-blocking medication may exacerbate asthma and other bronchospastic diseases, however, this effect may be minimised by the use of cardio-selective beta-blockers such as bisoprolol. Acarbose is an inhibitor of intestinal glucosi-dases (acting at the brush border) and may cause diarrhoea and loose stools due to the osmotic effect of a higher glucose load in the stool. Flatulence is also a side-effect reported by those taking acarbose due to the amount of glucose present in the colon available for metabolism by lower gastrointestinal organisms.

54 b. Lid retraction is a sign of sympathetic overactivity and can be seen in normal individuals who ingest large amounts of thyroxine with normal thyroid function. It can be used as a fairly reliable measure of the degree of treatment with thyroid-blocking medication. Hyperthyroidism is assessed clinically and confirmed biochemically with high levels of thyroid hormones (T4 and T3) and low levels of thyroid-stimulating hormone (TSH) due to negative feedback. The normal thyroid produces

T4 and T3 as driven by TSH from the pituitary, which in turn is driven by hypothalamic thyroid-releasing hormone (TRH). T4 is produced in abundance relative to T3, however, T3 is 4 times more metabolically active than T4 and is converted from T4 in peripheral tissues. Symptomatic control of hyperthyroidism is achieved acutely with beta-blockade such as propranolol until thyroid-blocking agents such as propylthiouracil or carbimazole have taken effect. This usually occurs over a period of weeks and therapy must be monitored in this period with regular tests of thyroid activity until a stable dosage regime has been established.

Beta-blockade is not usually required as long-term therapy if control of overactivity can be managed medically or surgically with subtotal or total thyroidectomy (if refractory to medical treatment).

55 e. In this gentleman with a history of peripheral vascular disease an exercise tolerance test would provide inadequate information. A thallium cardiac scan can assess the heart without putting pressure on the peripheral vasculature. The results of an ETT can be influenced by pain from intermittent claudication and therefore the thallium scan is a better alternative for risk stratification in this patient. The gold standard for investigation in this case is a coronary angiogram. It allows the vasculature of the heart to be visualised with ease and any obvious lesions may be managed at the same time, providing a relief from symptoms.

56 a. Both verapamil and diltiazem are calcium channel blockers.

They block calcium entry into the cell and its utilisation within the cell. They relax the coronary arteries and reduce the force of left ventricular contraction, which in turn reduces oxygen demand.

Diltiazem has a negative chronotropic effect which helps alleviate the symptoms of angina as will regular long-acting nitrates.

57 b. Warfarin is not indicated in the immediate management of myocardial infraction (MI). The anti-platelet effect of aspirin and clopidogrel has been shown to be beneficial in the treatment of MI.

58 e. New-onset atrial fibrillation should ideally be converted to sinus rhythm by DC cardioversion. DC cardioversion may precipitate systemic emboli from intracardiac thrombus. To avoid thromboembolic events, formal anticoagulation is required for a month before and after the cardioversion, unless:

• The arrhythmia is of less than 72 hours standing.

• No intracardiac thrombus is apparent on trans-oesophageal echocardiography.

Co-ordinated atrial activity may not resume for 2 weeks following cardioversion even if sinus rhythm is apparent on the ECG, for this reason anticoagulation should continue for 1 month usually in the form of warfarin. In this case it is inappropriate to start conservative medical management since the atrial fibrillation is of new onset (past 72 hours is cut off for cardioversion).

59 c. PTCA is the most appropriate management option for this gentleman. PTCA restores artery patency in more than 90% of patients. PTCA has fewer bleeding complications and recurrent ischaemia when compared to thrombolysis, however, a major drawback of PTCA is the need for 24-hour availability of an angioplasty suite and staff. The time for treatment is longer for patients receiving primary PTCA as compared to those receiving thrombolysis but if the facilities are available it is the preferred treatment option. None of the other options listed above are appropriate in the management of this case.

60 b. Contraindications to thrombolysis include:

• Known active bleeding source (e.g. peptic ulcer, active dyspepsia).

• Active menstruation.

• Cerebrovascular accident within 3 months.

• Surgery or head injury within last 3 months.

• Severe hypertension:

– Systolic more than 200 mmHG or diastolic more than 100 mmHg.

– Must be sustained (e.g. not responding to i.v. nitrates).

• Hypotension:

– Systolic less than 90 mmHg and not corrected by atropine (if bradycardia) or other rhythm correction.

• Chest trauma due to prolonged cardiac massage – if CPR more than 5 minutes assess risks with senior staff.

• On warfarin.

• Known or suspected aortic aneurysm.

• Known sensitivity to streptokinase or prior administration within last 24 months (for streptokinase administration only).

Extended matching questions

61 h. HSP is usually seen between the ages of 2 and 11 but approximately a quarter of cases may present in adulthood.

HSP commonly presents with a diffuse purpuric rash over thelower limbs and buttocks that can often be mistaken for non-accidental injury in a young child (hence the incorrect and improper involvement of social services on admission to hospital) associated with abdominal pain, vomiting and oedema.

Joint pain is also a common presenting feature and bloody stool indicated gastrointestinal involvement. The pathology is one of a small-vessel vasculitis with immune complex deposition in the vessels thus predictably leading to glomerular inflammation and signs of glomerulonephritis. About half of those presenting with HSP describe a preceding upper respiratory infection although many other putative triggers have been postulated.

Treatment is supportive and usually requires admission to hospital for monitoring of renal and gastrointestinal complications. Resolution is the rule but corticosteroids have been trialled to ameliorate symptoms.

62 b. IgA nephropathy (Berger's disease) is the commonest cause of glomerulonephritis worldwide – it is seen much more prevalently in Asian as compared to other populations. Berger's disease typically affects males more commonly than females and those in their twenties and thirties. The usual clinical presentation is with haematuria, which may be recurrent, usually following an upper respiratory tract infection. Less than 1 in 20 cases will present with acute renal failure and the nephrotic syndrome but spontaneous resolution does occur. An association with conditions such as gluten enteropathy and respiratory tract infections has led to the hypothesis that mucosal dysfunction is likely to play an important part in the development of the disease. Renal biopsy is the only modality to reliably diagnose IgA nephropathy and mesangial deposition of IgA and C3 seen on immunofluorescence is pathognomonic of the condition. Prognostically between 20% and 40% of all patients will eventually progress to end-stage renal failure (ESRF) requiring renal replacement therapy or transplantation.

63 a. Minimal change disease is the commonest cause of glomerulonephritis in children and can be difficult to distinguish from post-streptococcal glomerulonephritis as both can be brought on by preceding upper respiratory tract infections. An association in adults is with Hodgkin's lymphoma and this should be considered in adult patients presenting with signs of hypertension, proteinuria and oedema in whom a diagnosis of minimal change disease is considered. Renal biopsy should only be considered in children when tissue diagnosis is likely to alter management strategies and most renal physicians favour a therapeutic trial with corticosteroids with renal biopsy in more resistant cases. Histology by definition under light microscopy demonstrates little or no change thus electron microscopy is relied upon to look for subtle changes in foot process (podocyte) anatomy with podocyte fusion and retraction being the most common pathology.

64 i. Systemic lupus erythematosus is a systemic autoimmune condition with multi-organ involvement. Vasculitis is the underlying component that ties much of the organ dysfunction together with renal involvement predicting a poorer prognosis. Characteristically exhibiting the malar rash (butterfly rash so-called because of the double-winged appearance on either side of the nose) with a spectrum of symptoms ranging from neuropsychiatric to pulmonary, SLE can be difficult to diagnose unless it is borne in mind. Immune complex deposition of immunoglobulins directed against nuclear elements causes a glomerulonephritis often referred to as lupus nephritis with features on light microscopy graded by the WHO from I to VI.

Wire-loop lesions are seen in Grade IV microscopic appearances and are due to hyaline deposits. Treatment is directed at medically stabilising the patient until such time that they may require more definitive treatment of renal compromise such as replacement therapy or transplantation. Corticosteroids are the first-line therapy for all but severe renal disease at which point immunosuppressive agents such as azathioprine and cyclo-phosphamide improve renal function more significantly.

65 e. RPGN can manifest with a variety of conditions such as the systemic vasculitides, other systemic autoimmune conditions such as SLE, Goodpasture's disease, rheumatoid arthritis and glomerulonephritides of unknown or infectious aetiology.

Malignancy and drug therapy such as penicillamine and anti-tuberculous drugs can also cause a florid glomerulonephritis.

As the name suggests the decline in renal function to a level where intervention is required can be very rapid occurring anywhere from days/weeks at most aggressive to a few months.

Therefore early medical therapy is key in trying to influence the course of disease. Pathological correlates on renal histology are primarily of fibrinoid necrosis with crescent formation seen in over half the specimens biopsied.

66 c. Multi-infarct dementia (vascular dementia) usually presents in patients who have suffered multiple cerebrovascular events such as transient ischaemic attacks or strokes. Typically there is a step-wise deterioration of cerebral function with each event and relatives will often remark that the patient never recovered to the level he/she was before the stroke. Multi-infarct dementia accounts for about 25% of all strokes and should be considered in those with a history of cerebrovascular disease with global impairment of cognition.

67 g. Lewy-body dementia, as the name suggests, is characterised by the presence of Lewy bodies in the brainstem and cortex with a myriad of features of dementia and Parkinsonism. The difficulty in treating patients with this dementia is that using traditionalanti-parkinsonian drugs may lead to delusions, which themselvesare a common finding in dementia, and using neuroleptic drugs to counter delusions will worsen features of parkinsonism.

68 a. Alzheimer's dementia should be suspected in adults who demonstrate long-lasting problems with spatial navigation and visual awareness usually manifest as wandering or becoming lost. The mini-mental state examination is a relatively sensitive tool for screening for dementia but an ideal diagnosis requires exclusion of other reversible causes of dementia along with neuroimaging and histology. Found more commonly with increasing age there is evidence that 20% of those over 80 years old have dementia with many people with Down's syndrome manifesting signs of dementia earlier than 40 years of age.

69 h. Pseudo-dementia is a psychiatric illness that can mimic the apparent cognitive decline of true dementia. It is linked to depression and will characteristically ameliorate once the depression has been treated. The mini-mental state examination is not as sensitive a test for dementia in these cases as motivation plays a large part in determining a representative score. Clues to the diagnosis tend to come from the patient's affect and mood, however, as with any apparent dementia, it is important never to ascribe a reduction in cognition to pseudo-dementia without ruling out any organic cause of pathology.

70 e. This patient is too young to fit into the typical patterns of dementia and thus it is important that all organic causes for his behaviour be explored. The patient's nationality has an important bearing on narrowing down possible diagnoses and in a patient from Sub-Saharan Africa it is important to consider whether the patient's HIV status is a factor. More importantly, however, is to consider whether knowledge of HIV status is likely to alter the management strategy.

71 i. Haemophilia A and B and von Willebrand's disease may manifest as

223

bleeding from the gastrointestinal tract, mucous membranes, into joints and from any wounds (including surgical wounds). von Willebrand's disease is the most common inherited coagulopathy and results from either a reduction or lack of von Willebrand factor (vWF) or abnormally functioning vWF. vWF is involved in platelet function thus manifests in laboratory studies as an increase in bleeding time, high APTT with a normal INR.

Haemophiliacs are much more likely to exhibit major bleeding than von Willebrand's disease sufferers and bleeding into joints after trauma or exercise and into muscle after intramuscular injections are more commonly seen. The haemophilias are caused by a deficiency of factor VIII (haemophilia A) and factor IX (Christmas disease, haemophilia B) and behave clinically similarly. It should always be borne in mind when considering the differential diagnosis of any cause of bleeding that general bleeding diatheses may be responsible.

72 d. Haemorrhoids (or piles) are congested vascular cushions that aid the anal sphincter mechanism in maintaining continence. It is postulated that poor dietary fibre and straining at stool may contribute to the increase in rectal venous pressure that may precipitate haemorrhoid formation but mechanical factors such as rectal carcinoma, pelvic tumours and pregnancy all predispose to haemorrhoids. Typically bleeding is bright red and painless unless a prolapsed haemorrhoid becomes trapped in the sphincter or thrombosed. Sometimes patients have a sensation that something is descending in the rectum and may actually be able to feel prolapsed haemorrhoids. These are termed second-degree when they reduce spontaneously (first-degree haemorrhoids do not prolapse) and third-degree when they remain prolapsed.

Sclerotherapy, banding or surgical removal form the mainstay of treatment measures.

73 a. Angiodysplasia may be clinically asymptomatic or present with rectal bleeding; either occult in nature or associated with life-threatening haemorrhage. Due to their frequency in the elderly as opposed to young population the diagnosis is often only made at colonoscopy or mesenteric angiography. Angiodysplasia refers to vascular abnormalities, usually of veins, and are most commonly found in the caecum or ascending colon. Treatment is restricted to hemicolectomy if bleeding is severe or recurrent or if lesions are small or solitary then a trial of electrocoagula-tion during colonoscopy may be of benefit.

74 b. Osler–Weber–Rendu syndrome (hereditary haemorrhagic telangiectasia) is an autosomal-dominant disease involving dilatation of small arterioles and capillaries causing an increased tendency to bleed. Anticoagulation and anti-platelet agents

224

should be avoided if the syndrome is diagnosed. At one end of the spectrum small red blanching lesions are found on skin, mucous membranes and the gastrointestinal tract but at the other end the syndrome has been associated with the development of hepatic and pulmonary arteriovenous fistulas leading to high-output heart failure, cerebral embolism and cerebralabscesses. Recurrent epistaxis and gastrointestinal bleeds are the most common presentation of Osler–Weber–Rendu syndrome although stroke and cerebral abscess in young patients should always alert the clinician to the possibility of this disease.

75 f. Mesenteric embolus is a difficult diagnosis to make due to the myriad of insidious causes of rectal bleeding. The presentation of shock may be a feature of both hypovolaemia and infarction of bowel leading rapidly to faecal peritonitis and overwhelming sepsis if not caught early. Atrial fibrillation, bruit or other risk factors for thromboembolism may aid in pointing the surgeon to the right diagnosis. A careful history may reveal preceding symptoms of intermittent pain on eating and resultant weight loss due to reduction in blood flow through the mesenteric system, however, this is often uncommon in acute-on-chronic cases with the development of good collateral supply in the gastrointestinal tract even in the face of marked blockage. Resection of the necrotic bowel with either primary anastomosis or secondary closure of colostomy depending on site, age and co-morbidities is often the only treatment available at emergency presentation.

76 a. In the post-operative patient there are several potential causes of fever and shortness of breath. In this situation the answer is atelectasis. In the first 24 hours post-operatively this is most likely to be the cause of any shortness of breath or fever.

In the first 2–3 days pneumonia is more likely to be the cause.

In either case it is important to confirm the diagnosis by sending off blood tests, blood cultures and requesting a chest X-ray.

77 f. This gentleman has suffered a massive pulmonary embolus, which culminated in cardiac arrest. With his history of being treated for an embolus during the resuscitation streptokinase was administered although unfortunately, despite 3 cycles of resuscitation, this gentleman showed no signs of improving. As advised on the advanced life support course during a cardiac arrest reversible causes should be sought including:

• Hypokalaemia/hyperkalaemia.

• Hypothermia.

- Hypoxia.

- Hypovolaemia.

- Tension pneumothorax.

- Toxicity (drugs).

- Thromboembolism.

- Tamponade.

By working through these potential causes of cardiac arrest it is possible to treat those reversible causes effectively. During every cardiac arrest call that you attend you should always be thinking about the cause for each particular case as that quick thinking can be lifesaving.

78 c. This gentleman has suffered an aspiration pneumonia secondary to a stroke. If patients are not carefully monitored by the nursing staff they may continue to eat and drink despite having altered neurological status. If a patient's ability to swallow is impaired then they can develop aspiration pneumonia.

The commonest part of the lung to be affected by an aspiration pneumonia is the right lower lobe, this is due to the angulation of the right main bronchus meaning that food or any aspirate will preferentially end up there. Presentation of an aspiration pneumonia is identical to that of a normal pneumonia although the history may vary, the key difference is in the management. Aspiration pneumonia will require coverage for organisms normally found in the gastrointestinal tract, usually cefuroxime and metronidazole.

79 b. Given the details in the history it is sensible to be suspicious of a malignancy. Although this lady is young it is not uncommon for malignancies to present in this age group. She is complaining of a gradually worsening shortness of breath with a long history of cigarette smoking. The clinical findings of an effusion fit with the diagnosis of a lung cancer and analysis of the fluid would show an exudate with greater than 30 g/L of protein and presence of malignant cells. Whilst other causes of pleural effusions should be considered the presence of malignant cells confirms the diagnosis and further imaging tests should be carried out to confirm the location and subgroup of the cancer.

80 e. This scenario is clearly describing an exacerbation of COPD.

These are commonly caused by concurrent infection. In this case it appears that omission of her inhalers has resulted in reduced lung function and an opportunist infection has exacerbated the problem. With this subgroup of patients it is important to ensure that the infection is treated and that they are back on their usual bronchodilators and steroids before discharge in order to optimise their chances of coping once discharged. It is always important that appropriate follow-up arrangements are made to prevent similar episodes occurring in the future.

81 a. Appendicitis is both one of the easiest surgical conditions to diagnose and simultaneously one of the most difficult. The classical presentation of a young male or female with central colicky abdominal pain associated with nausea and vomiting, which subsequently localises to the right iliac fossa (with local peritoneal involvement) causing rebound tenderness and guarding leaves little else on the list of differentials. However, the variable position of the appendix and often relatively uncharacteristic presentation can often cause diagnostic conundrums. It must be heeded that torsion of the testis may present with the same clinical findings as appendicitis and there are cases of missed necrotic testes that were only discovered on the table when preparing the patient for appendicectomy. The abdominal examination must always include examination of the external genitalia, hernial orifices and consideration of digital rectal examination.

82 c. Diverticulitis is often colloquially referred to as the 'left-sided appendicitis'. It presents with many of the features of appendicitis: nausea, vomiting, rebound tenderness and guarding and localised pain in the left iliac fossa. The sigmoid colon is the unhappy recipient of the brunt of gastrointestinal disease for reasons still unknown and diverticulitis is most commonly found here. Terminology in diverticular disease is precise and should be used correctly:

- *Diverticulosis*: diverticula that are present and asymptomatic.

- *Diverticular disease*: refers to symptomatic diverticula.

- *Diverticulitis*: active inflammation of diverticula.

- *Complicated diverticulitis*: the presence of complications of diverticulitis, e.g. fistula, abscess or perforation.

The Hinchey classification grades perforated diverticulitis from Stage 1 to 4 depending on the extent of peritoneal contamin-ation and forms a useful guide to the severity of diverticulitis complication.

83 i. Rectosigmoid carcinoma may present with local, general or metastatic features. A change in bowel habit, large bowel obstruction, perforation, stricture or fistula associated with fresh rectal bleeding may all occur. General features associated with cancer are malaise, weight loss, a pyrexia of unknown origin (PUO) caused by activation or inflammatory cytokines and anaemia. As a rough guide right-sided tumours are more inclined to cause large bowel obstruction whilst those presenting on the left side (e.g. caecal carcinoma may present purely with an anaemia). Any unexplained anaemia or episode of rectal bleeding in older patients merits outpatient investigation such as colonoscopy if there is any suspicion of malignancy. More recently there has been a national initiative to introduce a colon cancer screening programme similar to that already in place for breast and cervical cancer screening and is planning to employ home faecal occult blood testing as part of the process.

84 f. Epigastric pain, vomiting and features of peritonism should alert the clinician to the possibility of a perforated peptic ulcer.

Risk factors for ulceration include drug therapy especially NSAIDs and steroids, smoking, excess alcohol intake, presence of *Helicobacter pylori* organism, severe burns (Curling's ulcer), acute stress reaction (Cushing's ulcer) and Zollinger–Ellison syndrome.

Perforation is investigated by both clinical examination and erect chest radiograph. Air under the diaphragm can help to confirm clinical suspicion and is present in more than 70% of cases of perforation.

85 b. Pancreatitis can be a complication of a myriad of causes.

These are best summarised by the mnemonic 'GET SMASHED' standing for **G**allstones, **E**thanol, **T**rauma, **S**teroids, **M**umps, **A**utoimmune disease, **S**corpion venom, **H**yperlipidaemia (also hypertension, hypercalcaemia, and hypothermia), **E**RCP and **D**rugs (rarely but significantly HMG-CoA reductase inhibitors ('statins') and anti-epileptic medication). Surgical signs associated with pancreatitis are the oft-quoted but rarely seen Grey-Turner's sign (bruising discolouration in the flanks) and Cullen's sign (bruising discolouration around the umbilicus).

Reactive pleural effusions can occur secondary to systemic inflammatory response evoked by severe pancreatitis and can be significant enough to affect the respiratory system.

86 g. It is important to remember that children are not simply small adults. There are a range of conditions that are specific to children and as a result their baseline observations vary.

Age (years)

Respiratory rate

Heart rate (bpm)

Systolic BP (mmHg)

(breaths per minute)

↕1 30–40

110–160 70–90

1–2 25–35

100–150 80–95

2–5 25–30

95–140 80–100

5–12 20–25

80–120

90–110

12 15–20

60–100 100–120

87 c. By the age of 9 months it is expected that a child will be able **262**

to sit up unaided. In all of these cases gestational age needs to be taken into account and any pre-term births need to have allowances made when assessing for normal development.

Between the ages of 13 and 18 months it is expected that a child will be able to walk unaided.

88 a. The vaccination schedule in the United Kingdom starts at the age of 2 months. At 2, 3 and 4 months infants are immunised against diphtheria, tetanus, pertussis, polio, *Haemophilus influenza B* and meningitis C. At the age of 12–15 months children are immunised against measles, mumps and rubella (MMR).

Between the ages of 3 and 5 years booster doses of diptheria, tetanus, pertussis, polio and MMR are administered. The next step in the schedule is the BCG aged 10–14 which provides approximately 75% protection against tuberculosis and the final step is a booster dose of diptheria, tetanus and polio aged approximately 18 years old.

89 a. This is a presentation of acute bronchiolitis. It is most commonly seen in those children under the age of 6 weeks or in those with chronic respiratory, cardiac or neurological deficits.

The commonest causative organism is the respiratory syncitial virus which accounts for 75% of cases. Those infants in respiratory distress may require non-invasive ventilation in the acute phase in addition to inhaled bronchodilators and there is some evidence for the use of ribavirin; a nucleoside analogue. Long-term consequences may include an obstructive bronchiolitis.

90 a. By 6–8 weeks it is believed that babies are able to follow movements with their eyes. At this age experts belies that their eyesight is developing and their vision extends up to a distance of approximately 30 cm. This is one of the reasons that babies are believed to form a strong bond with their mother as they can focus their gaze on them whilst feeding.

www.ingramcontent.com/pod-product-compliance
Lightning Source LLC
Chambersburg PA
CBHW031838170526
45157CB00001B/347